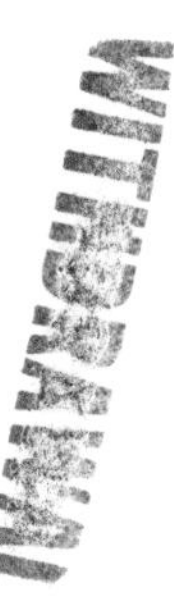
WITHDRAWAL

# Evaluating Health Maintenance Organizations

# Evaluating Health Maintenance Organizations

## A GUIDE FOR EMPLOYEE BENEFITS MANAGERS

PERRY MOORE

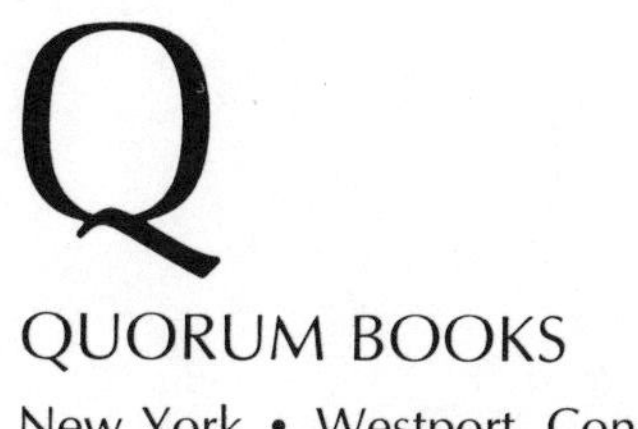

QUORUM BOOKS
New York • Westport, Connecticut • London

**Library of Congress Cataloging-in-Publication Data**

Moore, Perry.
Evaluating health maintenance organizations : a guide for employee benefits managers / Perry Moore.
p. cm.
Includes bibliographical references and index.
ISBN 0–89930–557–1 (alk. paper)
1. Health maintenance organizations—Evaluation. I. Title.
RA413.M66 1991
362.1'0425—dc20 91–4719

British Library Cataloguing in Publication Data is available.



Library of Congress Catalog Card Number: 91–4719
ISBN: 0–89930–557–1

First published in 1991

Quorum Books, One Madison Avenue, New York, NY 10010
An imprint of Greenwood Publishing Group, Inc.

Printed in the United States of America

The paper used in this book complies with the Permanent Paper Standard issued by the National Information Standards Organization (Z39.48–1984).

10 9 8 7 6 5 4 3 2 1

# Contents

# Tables

# Preface

Today there are nearly six hundred health maintenance organizations (HMOs) in the United States enrolling over 33 million Americans. The rapid growth of these alternative delivery organizations during the 1980s signaled their growing importance in America's battle to control health care costs. With HMOs emphasis on prepayment for comprehensive medical care, and their use of risk-sharing with providers to control costs, they represent a distinct divergence from traditional fee-for-service medicine.

Historically, providers of medical care have been paid a fee for each service which thus encouraged the delivery of more and more services. In contrast, HMOs are paid to deliver most health care services to an enrolled population for a particular period of time. Thus, HMOs' incentives are distinctly different from the traditional provider in fee-for-service medicine.

This book reviews the growth and development of HMOs in America throughout the 1970s and 1980s. HMOs' ability to control health care costs receives considerable attention. Of course, the danger in any attempt to reduce health care costs is that the quality of health care will suffer. Therefore, this book also gives much attention to the quality of care in HMOs.

Since employee health care costs now equal employers' after tax profits, employers and benefit managers may be particularly interested in this book. HMOs have significant potential to reduce health care costs if they are used properly by employers. Therefore, this book's numerous descriptions of HMO characteristics that are related to cost savings and quality control are useful when employers decide which HMOs to offer and recommend to their employees.

I am particularly indebted to my administrative assistant, Sue Sarner, whose efficiency, organizational prowess, and patience made this work possible. Furthermore, I must thank my wife, Marianne, who on more than a few occasions was patient with my frustrations in completing this project.

# 1

# The Health Care Crisis and HMOs

## INCREASING HEALTH CARE COSTS AND DECREASING SATISFACTION WITH CARE

Rising health care costs have consumed one-fifth of the economic growth in the United States between 1980 and 1987 (Citizens Fund 1990). During the same time, health care cost increases have eliminated nearly all real income growth for median income households in the United States. In 1987, per capita health spending in the United States was $2,050, which reflects a seven-fold increase since 1970. While health care expenditures consumed just over 7 percent of the GNP in 1970, they consumed over 11 percent of the GNP in 1987. Thus, health care costs have been increasing much more rapidly than general inflation.

Although these expenditures when considered in isolation are disturbing, when they are compared with expenditures of our major national competitors (Japan, Germany, France, Britain, and Canada), they are alarming. In 1987, the average per capita expenditures for these other nations ($1,069) was approximately half of U.S. expenditures. The United States spends 124 percent more per capita for health care than does Japan, and 91 percent more than Germany.

This discrepancy in national expenditures means that U.S. companies are spending more than their international competitors, which increases the price of U.S. products and decreases their competitiveness in international markets. For example, over $700 of the price of Chrysler Corporation autos pay for health care for Chrysler employees in the United States. In comparison, only $220 of the price of Canadian-made automobiles are for health care costs. If health care costs had consumed the same level of real economic growth in the United States as in Japan and Germany, the United States would have had over $70 billion more per year to invest in plant expansion, research, and development (Citizens Fund 1990).

From 1965 to 1987, health spending by businesses doubled as a proportion of fringe benefits reaching 41 percent in 1987, and equaled 7 percent of wages and salaries. The ratio of health spending to after-tax corporate profits increased from 14 percent in 1965 to around 94 percent in the 1980s (Levit et al. 1989). Thus, with health care costs equaling profits, it is apparent why employers are becoming much more concerned about containing health care costs.

If these increases in health care costs were accompanied by corresponding increases in quality and satisfaction, perhaps the expenditures would be more palatable. Unfortunately, this is not the case. The United States infant mortality rate is twenty-second in the world and double that of Japan. Similarly, the United States ranks twenty-first in child mortality. Finally, it ranks twelfth in life expectancy, while Japan ranks number one (Citizens Fund 1990).

Americans are apparently much less satisfied than are citizens of other nations with their health care. Recent Gallup polls indicate that among ten major industrialized countries, Americans and Italians are most upset with their health care systems (Blendon et al. 1990). So although the United States spends the most per capita for health care, it does not rank at the top in national health statistics or in citizen satisfaction.

## CONTROLLING HEALTH CARE COSTS: REGULATION VERSUS COMPETITION

There are two basic approaches to controlling health care cost increases—regulation and competition. Most of the other major industrialized nations use regulation much more extensively than the United States. For example, in Great Britain the government owns the hospitals and pays capitated payments (lump sums paid for all health care received by an individual during a specified time period) to general practitioners. Thus, health care delivery is highly regulated in Britain. In France, Germany, the Netherlands, and Canada, the governments, through their national sick funds, negotiate rates with both hospitals and doctors. Thus, government regulation of health care is extensive in these nations.

The United States has also tried some regulatory approaches. We have used health system agencies as planning bodies for regional health care delivery. During the early 1970s, government attempted to control hospital and physician charges through the economic stabilization program. One of the most far-reaching regulatory actions by the government has been Medicare's prospective payment system which establishes a payment rate for each diagnostic related group of services.

Of course, federal and state governments have regulated health care in order to raise standards and assure safety and quality. For example, states license physicians, nurses, and other medical professionals. Government funding of medical education also regulates entry into various medical professions. New drugs and medical devices must obtain the approval of the Food and Drug

Administration before they can be used extensively. States also require insurers to maintain reserves to pay beneficiaries.

While the United States has engaged in significant regulation of Americans' health care, the nation has generally depended on competition to structure the delivery of medical care and to control its costs. This results in large measure from our free-market tradition and the entrepreneurial values of our culture. Health care providers have utilized appeals to this tradition to discourage and defeat attempts to promote more government regulation of fees and rates. Moreover, providers have warned that government regulation could undermine individuals' freedom to select providers, interfere in doctor-patient relationships, and undermine quality of care. Thus, those who believe in competition assume that liberty and the public good result from individual initiatives with decentralized decision-making and a limited role for government (Altman and Rodwin 1988).

### Competition in Health Care Markets

Competition within health care markets is markedly dissimilar to competition in other markets. These dissimilarities compromise the health market's ability to control demand and prices. The demand for medical care tends to be inelastic. In other words, the demand for health care tends to remain strong regardless of the price of such care. If one is sick, one wants to get well even if the care is quite expensive. Thus, as prices increase, demand does not necessarily decrease.

Perhaps the biggest difference between health care markets and other markets is that those who consume health care often do not pay for it. In 1965, governments (federal, state, and local) paid for approximately 20 percent of all health care (Levit et al. 1989). By 1988, the proportion had increased to 31 percent. Likewise, in 1965 employers paid just over 22 percent of all health expenditures. By 1987, the employers' share had increased to 28 percent. Thus, in 1987, government and employers paid almost 60 percent of all health care expenses. Obviously, if one does not pay for a highly valued good (health care), then one will consume more of it.

Even that portion of health care purchased by individuals often is paid through insurance premiums. In other words, patients make relatively few direct payments to their providers as they consume health care. In 1965, patients paid over 48 percent of all costs through direct payments. However, this decreased to just over 25 percent in 1987 (Levit et al. 1989). If consumers pay for services not as they use them, but through insurance premiums, then the cost of health care does not serve as a disincentive to its consumption. Indeed, the incentive is to consume even more since the insurance has already been purchased. In other words, why not use insurance and validate the wisdom behind its purchase?

Consumers of health care, unlike most consumers in other markets, have very little information about the quality, effectiveness and efficiency of the health products they purchase. Indeed, it has been said that Americans seek more information about purchasing an appliance or a car than they do for purchasing their own health care. Even if information is sought, however, it is not easily obtained. One does not find readily available data about physicians' practice patterns, malpractice history, and so on.

In the absence of complete information, consumers are likely to believe that more medical care equals better care. Of course, having most costs covered by payers other than the patient also encourages this conclusion. In addition, providers' economic self-interest as well as their professional ethics support ordering more services. Medicine involves a great amount of uncertainty and risk which physicians attempt to reduce by using more tests and offering more services. Likewise, doctors concerned about malpractice lawsuits tend to err on the side of too many services rather than too few. All of these tendencies undermine true competition and subvert the controlling influences of supply and demand in medical care markets.

Another major difference between health care markets and other markets is that the providers of health care can generate their own demand. Patients become very dependent upon the recommendations of their physicians. If the doctor recommends another visit or another test, the patient is generally unable to critically evaluate the recommendation and thus generally agrees with the physician.

It was hoped that as the physician supply increased, the unit price of physician services would be constrained as more and more physicians competed for the same number of patients. However, since physicians can generate demand for their own services, areas with large concentrations of doctors may generate more medical services per capita as the number of doctors increase. Moreover, physician's fees have not declined even as the supply of physicians has increased dramatically. In fact, physicians fees continued to outpace the general rate of inflation throughout most of the 1980s (Fuchs and Hahn 1990).

As a result of the above dynamics, competition in health care markets is often characterized by competition in quality, or what is often confused with quality, rather than competition in costs. Quality is often defined as new technologies and procedures, new equipment, attractive offices, and amenities, and so on. Of course, this type of competition tends to increase rather than decrease costs.

## HMOs, COMPETITION, AND QUALITY

At least in theory, health maintenance organizations (HMOs) should counter many of the anti-competitive elements in health care markets. While there are many kinds of HMOs, they usually share some common elements. They serve defined populations of enrollees who receive comprehensive health care from HMOs in return for a prepaid amount for each enrollee.

The prepayment is critical in that it tends to counterbalance the inflationary tendencies of fee-for-service (FFS). Under FFS, doctors and hospitals are paid according to a fee for each service. Hence, as the number of services increase, the costs increase. Obviously, it is in the providers' economic self-interest to increase services. On the other hand, HMOs receive revenue from enlisting more enrollees rather than offering more individual services. Indeed, HMOs have real incentives to decrease utilization in order to conserve revenues.

With prepayment, HMOs assume much of the risk in offering health care to a specific population. Therefore, it is in HMOs' interest to keep their enrollees healthy and out of the hospital. In theory, HMOs would compete on the size of the prepayment. As a result, more cost competition would be injected into health care markets.

HMOs' potential to encourage competition and constrain costs appealed to the conservative philosophy of the Nixon Administration in the early 1970s. Thus, in the HMO Act of 1973, the federal government actively encouraged the development of HMOs as a way to control health care cost increases. Chapter 2 describes the early history of prepaid group plans as well as the specifics of the HMO Act of 1973.

The capacity of HMOs to control costs and encourage competition depends on the specific kinds and characteristics of HMOs. There are four major types of HMOs—staff, group, network, and independent practice associations. These are described in Chapter 2 as are the more recent developments of HMOs and the typical benefits and premiums found in HMOs.

The chief way in which HMOs control costs is reducing utilization. Chapter 3 discusses the various methods that different types of HMOs use to reduce utilization and reviews research on HMOs' capacity to lower use of health care services.

Reductions in utilization should logically lead to reductions in costs. Cost studies of HMOs versus fee-for-service plans are compared in Chapter 3. Do HMOs achieve a one-time cost reduction in health care costs, or do they continue to build on one year's savings with even more savings in subsequent years? This question is explored with an examination of trends in HMO costs versus FFS costs in Chapter 3.

HMOs could reduce costs through greater efficiency as well as through reductions in utilization. In other words, an HMO might save money by delivering the same number of services with fewer resources. Thus, the ability of HMOs to deliver a unit of health care more efficiently or less expensively than FFS providers is explored in Chapter 3.

Many critics of HMOs say that HMOs only appear to save money. In fact, so these critics argue, HMOs attract a healthier group of enrollees (e.g., favorable selection) and so do not actually lower utilization and save costs. Rather, HMOs enroll those who need less health care. Since this criticism strikes at the very heart of the HMO concept, the problem of favorable selection into HMOs is extensively explored in Chapter 3. Since favorable selection could be influenced by both enrollment strategies and disenrollment, both topics receive attention.

Chapter 3 concludes with a general review of what steps employers can take to discourage and control the impact of favorable selection of their employees into HMOs.

While some critics of HMOs accept that HMOs may reduce utilization and costs, they claim that quality is also reduced as utilization is lowered. On the other hand, supporters of HMOs contend that there are structural elements within HMOs that promote quality. In theory, HMOs have formal organizational structures that, other things being equal, tend to require more interaction among colleagues and more peer review. These more organized relationships should provide greater continuity and coordination of care.

The quality of care in HMOs is reviewed in Chapter 4. Quality in health care is generally measured by structural measures (i.e., training, certification, staffing ratios, equipment), process measures (i.e., appropriate protocols for a particular diagnosis) or outcome measures (i.e., actual health status of patient). The quality of care in HMOs as measured by each of these approaches is compared to similar measures in the fee-for-service sector.

Of course, a critical dimension in any assessment of quality is the satisfaction of the patient. Therefore, consumer satisfaction with HMOs is also analyzed in Chapter 4. Since disenrollment can be a sign of consumer dissatisfaction, it is also reviewed. Any HMO seriously concerned about quality should have an effective quality assurance process. The essential components of a quality assurance process are also discussed in Chapter 4.

Since employers pay most of the premiums to HMOs, their satisfaction with HMOs is critical. In recent years, employers have had numerous complaints about HMOs. Most of these concern provisions of the original HMO Act of 1973 (e.g., dual-choice mandate, the rating requirements, the equal dollar contributions, and the federal qualification process). These concerns are discussed in Chapter 5 within the context of the 1988 amendments to the HMO Act.

Employers have the chief responsibility to assure that HMOs provide quality care as efficiently as possible. Chapter 5 emphasizes the importance of employer evaluation of HMOs. Important qualities of HMOs which employers should review include accessibility, benefits, rates, reputation, management, financial condition, enrollment procedures, medical services, and quality assurance and utilization review processes. Important factors that employers should review in each of these areas are described in Chapter 5.

The success and quality of any HMO depends on the ability, commitment, and courtesy of its physicians, and its relations with hospitals and other providers. The variability within the practice of medicine (e.g., different levels of treatment for similar diagnoses) allows considerable opportunity for HMOs to encourage their doctors to practice conservative medicine. Chapter 6 describes the methods that HMOs use to influence their physicians' behavior. These include both selective recruitment and carefully crafted orientation. HMOs also provide feedback to physicians concerning their individual behavior as compared to other physicians in the plan with the intent of changing physicians' behavior.

Chapter 6 provides extensive discussion of the financial arrangements that HMOs use to influence doctors' practice patterns. These compensation strategies include capitation, salaries, "withholds," and fee-for-service. Chapter 6 also describes those factors affecting the relationship between hospitals and HMOs. Competition in local hospital markets (e.g., number of hospitals, segmentation of the market, occupancy rates) directly affects HMOs' ability to negotiate favorable contracts with hospitals. This relationship between the local hospital market and HMO contracts is discussed in Chapter 6, as are the factors that limit HMOs' influence on hospitals. Moreover, the relationship between pharmacies and HMOs is reviewed in Chapter 6.

Since Medicaid and Medicare account for 10 percent of the entire federal budget, HMOs' ability to reduce the costs of these programs is of considerable concern. Chapter 7 investigates this topic as well as HMOs' capacity to address other problems in Medicare and Medicaid. In addition, the quality of care in Medicare and Medicaid HMOs is investigated as is the satisfaction of Medicare beneficiaries and Medicaid recipients with their HMOs.

Since numerous employers and employees are located in rural areas, and because rural areas often have more pronounced health problems than urban areas, the ease of developing HMOs in rural areas is assessed in Chapter 8. There are more significant problems in developing rural HMOs (i.e., smaller population base over which to spread capital costs). These are reviewed as are the factors in developing successful rural HMOs.

A primary competitor with HMOs is preferred provider organizations (PPOs). They differ from HMOs in that most do not involve prepayment, and they generally do not require risk-sharing by providers. These differences and others are detailed in Chapter 9. Also, methods used by PPOs to control costs are assessed. These are compared to cost control efforts in HMOs. Finally, employers' and employees' satisfaction with HMOs and PPOs are contrasted.

The conclusion stresses that competition as a general strategy to control health care costs will be effective only if employers act much more aggressively to prevent cost increases. HMOs must play a vital role in this more aggressive, competitive approach to health care. However, HMOs must develop their management information systems and be more responsive to employers' requests for information and experience-based ratings. Moreover, HMOs must develop much more risk-sharing by providers before doctors and hospitals will have the appropriate financial incentives to avoid overutilization.

HMOs may be the last best hope that a competitive approach can successfully control increases in health care costs. If HMOs cannot control such costs, the nation may move from the competitive strategy of controlling costs to a regulatory approach. Those who seek to avoid government domination of health care delivery should carefully consider HMOs' potential to control cost increases while also providing quality care.

2

# History and Development of HMOs

## EARLY PREPAID PRACTICE PLANS

While the term "health maintenance organization" was coined by Paul Ellwood in 1970, the concept of an HMO was built upon a long history of prepaid group practice (PGP) dating back to the 1920s and 1930s. Indeed, the idea of groups of physicians organizing to provide comprehensive health care to patients is as old as the Republic (Falkson 1979). However, group medical practice was not considered a serious alternative to solo practice until the founding of the Mayo Clinic in Rochester, Minnesota in 1883. Its success prompted the formation of similar groups in other large cities.

The modern movement of prepaid group practice plans originated in 1929 with the formation of the Ross-Loos Clinic in Los Angeles and the Elk City Cooperative in Elk City, Oklahoma. The Ross-Loos plan consisted of a group of physicians who contracted on a prepaid basis to deliver health care to the employees of the Los Angeles water department. The local medical society vigorously opposed the plan. While the Ross-Loos plan represented a threat to the medical profession from within, the Elk City Cooperative represented an even greater threat from outside—the consumers who controlled the plan (Falkson 1979). The Elk City Cooperative grew out of the harsh conditions of the depression and the need for low-cost health care in rural communities. The Elk City Cooperative hired salaried physicians to provide health care to members who paid a fixed-sum prepayment. From 1924 to 1954, the county and state medical societies of Oklahoma tried numerous ways to sabotage the plan. For example, the plan's physicians were ousted from the local medical society. Hospitals revoked their staffing privileges and attempts were made to revoke their medical licenses. In nearly all cases, the courts rejected these attempts to undermine group practice physicians.

Prior to 1932, the major method of financing medical care was the patient paying fees for services received. While such fees enhanced the professional autonomy of the provider, they became very unreliable during the depression. Doctors and hospitals had to find a way to reduce the uncertain cash flows of the fee-for-service system. The answer came in prepayment (Falkson 1979).

In 1932, the American Hospital Association adopted a prepayment plan that had been used by Baylor Hospital to halt the shrinkage of its revenues. From this plan emerged the first Blue Cross Plan. Blue Cross would eliminate the hospitals' and doctors' dependence on the fragile finances of patients by acting as a fiscal intermediary between patients and hospitals. By collecting fixed premiums for specific hospital benefits, and by reimbursing providers on the basis of costs incurred, Blue Cross provided an attractive way to solve critical economic problems without disrupting the practice patterns of physicians and hospitals (Falkson 1979). Increased costs were simply passed on to consumers as higher premiums, deductibles and copayments. On the other hand, the essence of the consumer-sponsored, cooperative health care plans was the shifting of economic risk to providers and hospitals. It should be clear why the medical profession preferred Blue Cross over the early PGPs.

Despite the strong opposition of the medical profession, the consumers' prepaid movement continued. In 1937, the Group Health Association was initiated by employees of the Homeowners Loan Corporation who sought to reduce the number of mortgage defaults by reducing the impact of catastrophic illness, the most prevalent source of foreclosures (Falkson 1979).

At about the same time, Kaiser Industries got involved in group health care delivery. Dr. Sidney Garfield and several other doctors had organized a group practice to serve the needs of construction workers who were building canal projects crossing Southern California. When Kaiser began the Grand Coulee Dam project in Washington, Garfield was asked to establish a prepaid group plan for Kaiser employees and their families. It is debatable whether the plan was set up to save money or to provide care that was otherwise unobtainable. Whatever the intent, the Kaiser plans did economize. Although Kaiser experienced some difficulty in recruiting medical staff in the early years, it turned the handicap into a virtue by consciously attempting to maintain lower levels of staffing than fee-for-service providers (Rayner 1988).

Kaiser replicated the Grand Coulee plan in other areas of the West Coast during World War II. These plans were merged under the Kaiser-Permanente Foundation. After the war, the program was opened to the general public. By 1954, the Kaiser plans were well established and increasing their enrollments all along the West Coast. Kaiser-Permanente used many of the principles that were later applied in other nonprofit prepaid plans including: group practice, integration of facilities, prepayment, and voluntary enrollment (Rayner 1988).

Other prepaid plans were developed by all kinds of organizations from labor unions to insurance companies. The Health Insurance Plan of New York (HIP) was initiated by Mayor Fiorello La Guardia for city employees in 1944; the Group Health Cooperative of Puget Sound was started by consumers in 1947; and the Community Health Association of Detroit was established in 1956 by the United Auto Workers. In the same year, the Group Health Mutual Insurance Company broke with tradition and offered direct prepaid health services, thereby indicating the potential interest of indemnity insurers in prepaid plans.

During the 1930s and 1940s, prepaid medicine faced persistent resistance from fee-for-service medicine. At the urging of state and local medical societies, twenty-two states had by 1971 enacted laws prohibiting the establishment of organizations to engage in "corporate medical practice, conjointly with non-physicians." However, the courts usually invalidated such laws (Falkson 1979).

Resistance to the success of the Kaiser plans took a more positive approach in the San Joaquin Valley of California in 1954. Local fee-for-service physicians sponsored an independent nonprofit foundation that would provide lower cost medical care for a prepaid amount. All community physicians who chose to participate agreed to accept the fee schedules of the foundation and peer review to assure the appropriateness of their practice patterns (Falkson 1979).

As physicians obtained more experience with the foundation, they adjusted their service patterns in accordance with the peer review criterion, and their fees were adjusted in reference to the fixed sum, prepayment pool of dollars collected as insurance premiums by the foundation (Falkson 1979). While the foundation sometimes had to pay reduced fees to keep the insurance pool solvent, the more typical experience was that the pool more than covered the fees and thus provided a year-end bonus to the participating physicians. Therefore, the physicians accepted the risk of discounted fees as well as the bonuses of efficiency. This foundation and others like it were the precursors to the modern Independent Practice Association (IPA) type of HMO.

## GOVERNMENT INVOLVEMENT IN HEALTH CARE

Although the U.S. Public Health Service had long been providing direct health services to wards of the federal government including Indians, Eskimos, and Aleuts, the delivery of personal medical services to the bulk of the U.S. population was held to be a private, not a public enterprise until the twentieth century. However, in 1935, the Social Security Act authorized federal grants-in-aid to the states for general public health programs and for maternal and child care (Falkson 1979). Likewise, the Farm Security Administration began to build health care programs for rural areas during the Depression and World War II.

Starting in 1936 with the National Cancer Act and escalating dramatically after the war, Congress appropriated millions to fight disease through basic and applied research. After the war, the federal government started the Hill Burton Health Facilities Construction Program which dramatically expanded hospital beds across the country. Indeed, by the early 1970s, there was an oversupply of 25 to 33 percent. During the 1960s, the federal government significantly expanded its role in health care delivery in the Medicaid and Medicare programs. Medicaid provided subsidized payments for health services to impoverished populations. Medicare also subsidized the demand side of the health care economy by providing payments for comprehensive health services for elderly citizens.

The impact of all these federal efforts between 1940 and 1970 increased demand for medical services, emphasized high cost care, and further fragmented health care delivery. Subsidies for the expansion of health facilities resulted in the overproduction of hospital beds. Biomedical and training grants encouraged excessive specialization and deterred development of community-based medical practice. Third-party payments to hospitals and specialists tended to bloat medicine's pricing structure while also decreasing consumer choice in the purchasing process and exaggerating the real need for health services. Medicare and Medicaid stimulated demand for primary and community-based medicine without expanding the supply of such services. In fact, federal policies supported the trend toward specialization and high cost technology. Thus, the federal subsidies "magnified and intensified the health system's internal contradictions" (Falkson 1979).

## BIRTH OF THE HMO CONCEPT

Because of the contradictions noted above and the high inflation of health care costs caused in part by these contradictions, the Nixon administration in 1969 was becoming more and more concerned about what was being called the "health care crisis." At the same time, Paul Ellwood, M.D., Executive Director of the American Rehabilitation Foundation, was concluding a comprehensive review of the health care system and possible ways of reforming it. In 1970, senior HEW officials asked Ellwood to share his suggestions for reforming the health care system. Although Ellwood was impressed with the economies of prepaid group practices and health care foundations or corporations over fee-for-service medicine, he also knew that no proposal which had been so vigorously opposed by organized medicine would have much chance of political success. Thus, he purposefully invented the neutral term "health maintenance organization." The term was explicitly calculated to be vague and neutral sounding (Rayner 1988).

"Health" rather than "medical" was used to emphasize prevention, early diagnosis and early treatment. "Maintenance" focused on maintaining health rather than treating illness (Falkson 1979). "Organization" was used instead of "corporation" or "group practice" because of medicine's longstanding opposition to these terms.

Ellwood's emphasis on decentralized independent health delivery organizations which would respond to the incentives of the market appealed to the conservative Nixon Administration. The proposal resisted direct governmental intervention in health care, which reduced opposition from organized medicine, and it promised to bring more business principals and incentives into health care, which appealed to conservatives and Republicans (Rayner 1988).

## THE HEALTH MAINTENANCE ORGANIZATION ACT OF 1973

The HMO Act of 1973 was designed to stimulate the growth of prepaid group practice. The act provided grants, loans and demonstration projects in an effort to stimulate interest in the HMO concept by both consumers and providers. The act also preempted many state laws put in place by local medical societies to obstruct the formation and development of prepaid group practice.

The act required employers with twenty-five or more employees who provided health insurance benefits to offer HMO coverage if a federally qualified HMO operated in the area. Thus, the law sought to provide HMOs more market access in areas where employers were reluctant to offer HMOs as part of their benefits program. The act also required the employer to contribute no less per person enrolled in the HMO than was contributed for each employee enrolled in the traditional health plans.

In order to be federally qualified, HMOs had to provide certain mandatory benefits, had to use community rating, were restricted in how much they could charge patients for out-of-pocket expenses, had to offer a thirty-day open enrollment period each year, had to offer quality assurance programs, and had to provide consumer participation and health education opportunities.

## TYPES OF HMOs

Although there are a number of different types of HMOs, all share certain generic characteristics. All HMOs serve a defined population of enrolled members. Subscriber enrollment is voluntary. Payments are made by the members or their employers for a specific period of time and made periodically. The HMO assumes a contractual responsibility to provide or assure the delivery of stated benefits. The HMO assumes at least part of the financial risk or gain from the delivery of health care.

Luft (1981) has noted that these generic characteristics of HMOs have important implications. The defined enrolled population allows HMOs to know to whom they must provide services. This is critical to planning. Voluntary enrollment implies competition among HMOs and between HMOs and other insurers and providers. If HMOs had a monopoly, their services might deteriorate and/or their prices increase.

The set prepayment is critical in the definition of HMOs. An HMO will gain no advantage by offering more services than needed. In fact, providing fewer services will produce more net revenue. Since HMOs assume some financial risk or gain in the provision of services, they also have a financial incentive to reduce excessive utilization.

While there are numerous types of HMOs and HMO hybrids, four main types tend to dominate the market: staff, group, network, and the independent practice associations (IPAs).

*Staff HMOs* are the classical prepaid group plan in which participating physicians are salaried employees of the HMO who generally see only HMOs' prepaid patients. Bonuses based on the performance of the plan may also be an important part of physician compensation. The HMO provides most outpatient services at its multispecialty ambulatory care center or centers. While some staff-model HMOs own their own hospitals, most contract with community hospitals.

*Group HMOs* contract with an independent group medical practice whose members become the HMOs' participating doctors. The group practice may have pre-dated the HMO and may previously have served fee-for-service patients. The HMO pays the group practice a capitated fixed sum for each enrollee per month. Referrals to doctors outside the group are also paid from the capitation. Profit and risk-sharing are generally important elements of compensation. Since bonuses or losses tend to reward physicians for individual and collective performance, there are similarities between staff-model and group-model HMOs.

*Network HMOs* closely resemble group-model HMOs except that the network HMO contracts with two or more independent group practices. The HMO makes capitation payments to each group for enrollees who select that group. Most groups in network HMOs continue to serve fee-for-service patients. However, more and more groups in networks are moving to capitation for hospital as well as physician services, or they share heavily in the risk subject to a maximum limit beyond which the HMO assumes responsibility (Fox and Heinen 1987).

*Independent Practice Associations* (IPAs) contract with HMOs to provide health care to HMO enrollees. While the enrollees or their employers pay a capitated fee to the HMO, the HMO contracts with the doctors in the IPA on a discounted fee-for-service basis with opportunity to recoup the discounted amount if a surplus remains at the end of the year. In some IPAs, doctors are not members of a separate organization at all, but contract directly with the HMO on a fee-for-service basis or per capita. Doctors who participate in the IPA may see both HMO and non-HMO patients and also may belong simultaneously to several competing IPAs. In such circumstances, the doctor's identification with an individual HMO may be relatively weak.

HMOs may also be classified as profit, non-profit, federally or nonfederally qualified and open or closed. Staff and group models are generally closed panels because their physicians see only HMO patients. On the other hand, network and IPA models are open panels in that participating physicians see both HMO and non-HMO patients.

HMOs may become federally qualified by applying to the Health Care Financing Administration. Federal qualification may be viewed as a positive endorsement or a sign of quality assurance by some employers. Only federally qualified HMOs can use the Health Maintenance Act of 1973 to mandate employers to offer at least one closed panel and one open panel HMO to employees.

Many HMOs do not seek federal qualification in order to maximize flexibility and to avoid the requirements necessary for qualification.

Recently, there has been a blurring of HMO organizational forms. Hybrid forms have developed incorporating features of several different types. For example, open-ended HMOs allow enrollees to receive services from non-HMO providers under a financing arrangement similar to traditional indemnity insurance. Benefits received outside the HMO are generally less comprehensive than those provided by the HMO providers, and deductibles and copayments are usually required.

These various types of HMOs exist along a managed care continuum from a managerially 'tight' arrangement based on HMO ownership of ambulatory facilities and hospitals, and HMO employment of doctors and other providers on salaries (staff-model HMOs), to ''loose'' arrangements (generally IPAs) that mix fee-for-service medicine, physician networks, and contracted care (Rayner 1988).

## DEVELOPMENT OF HMOs FROM 1973 TO 1989

In 1970, InterStudy identified thirty-seven HMOs in fourteen states with California having sixteen or 43 percent of the total (Gruber et al. 1988). HMOs were obviously most popular in the West where 67 percent of all HMOs were located. Only one was located in the South. Approximately three million people were enrolled in HMOs.

The HMO Act of 1973 accelerated the pace of HMO development by providing planning and development grants to qualified HMOs. From 1974 to 1980, the federal government provided over $190 million in grants and loans to HMOs. Private investment was considerable, estimated at $784 million prior to 1974 (Gruber et al. 1988). By 1975, over one hundred and seventy-five HMOs were in operation with estimated enrollments of nearly six million (see Table 2.1). Thus, the number of HMOs had increased by over five times and the enrollment had doubled since 1970.

Amendments to the HMO Act of 1973 liberalized requirements for federal qualification in 1976. As a result, there was more widespread industry acceptance of federal qualification and the number of such plans increased from forty-two in 1977 to seventy-nine in 1978 (Gruber et al. 1988).

From 1978 to 1980, enrollments in HMOs increased by over 33 percent to over nine million enrollees. However, in 1982 enrollment slowed. Perhaps this resulted from the high national unemployment (over 8.5 percent) that resulted in the loss of employer-sponsored health benefits for many employees.

From 1983 to 1987, HMOs enjoyed tremendous enrollment increases of 15 to 25 percent, and enrollment more than doubled from 12.5 million to over 28 million. Several reasons account for this growth. First, the HMO concept had become much more familiar to both consumers and employers. Second, HMO premiums had increased more slowly than those of traditional indemnity plans. By the mid-1980s, many HMO premiums were the same as or lower than the

**Table 2.1**
**Growth of HMOs**

| Year | Number of Plans | Enrollment (millions) |
|---|---|---|
| 1970 | 37 | 3.0 |
| 1974 | 142 | 5.3 |
| 1975 | 178 | 5.7 |
| 1976 | 175 | 6.0 |
| 1977 | 165 | 6.3 |
| 1978 | 203 | 7.5 |
| 1979 | 215 | 8.2 |
| 1980 | 236 | 9.1 |
| 1981 | 243 | 10.2 |
| 1982 | 265 | 10.8 |
| 1983 | 280 | 12.5 |
| 1984 | 306 | 15.1 |
| 1985 | 393 | 18.9 |
| 1986 | 595 | 23.7 |
| 1987 | 662 | 28.6 |
| 1988 | 653 | 30.3 |
| 1989 | 607 | 31.9 |
| 1990 | 575 | 33.1 |

*Sources*: Office of Health Maintenance Organizations, *National Census of Prepaid Health Plans* (Washington, DC: U.S. Department of Health, Education and Welfare, 1978, 1979, 1980); Group Health Association of America, *National HMO Census Survey, 1976-1977 Summary* (Washington, DC: GHAA, 1977); InterStudy, *National HMO Census* (Excelsior, MN: InterStudy, 1981-1984); InterStudy, *The InterStudy Edge* (Excelsior, MN: InterStudy, Spring, 1988); InterStudy, *The June 1985 HMO Summary* (Excelsior, MN: InterStudy, 1985); InterStudy, *The 1986 June Update* (Excelsior, MN: InterStudy, 1986); *InterStudy, The Bottom Line: HMO Premiums and Profitability: 1988-1989* (Excelsior, MN: InterStudy, 1989); and InterStudy, *The InterStudy Edge* (Excelsior, MN: InterStudy, Spring, 1990).

premiums charged by traditional plans. At the same time, the HMOs generally offered more comprehensive services. Third, HMOs had become more accepted by Wall Street and the major financial markets. This provided access to capital for many plans and encouraged the development of multiplan organizations (Wrightson 1990). Fourth, in areas where providers had strongly opposed HMOs, the opposition was beginning to crumble. Physicians sought access to IPAs in order to compete with staff-model and group-model HMOs and to maintain their patient loads as the supply of physicians increased.

By 1987, however, enrollment growth had slowed and the number of HMOs had declined. Reasons for the slower growth included (1) increased competition from other health care products, (2) employers' increasing dissatisfaction with HMOs' inability to use experience-based premiums, and (3) employers increasing frustrations with HMOs' inability to provide group-specific data on costs, use, and quality (Gruber et al. 1988).

## HMO ACT AMENDMENTS OF 1988

The 1988 Amendments to the HMO Act included several major changes concerning rate setting and the equal employer contributions to HMOs. Under the original HMO Act, federally qualified HMOs had to use community ratings when establishing premiums for employers. Thus, the HMOs total population's use of health care determined the rates charged an individual employer within the HMO. However, many employers believed that their healthier employees were being disproportionately attracted to HMOs. Hence, they believed their employees were healthier than the average person in the HMO. Therefore, employers sought experience-based ratings or ratings based on the actual health care experience of their particular employees. The 1988 HMO Act Amendments provide for more flexible experience-based, prospective rate setting.

Under the original HMO Act, employers had to make contributions to mandated HMOs that were equal in dollars to those provided to other indemnity insurance companies or to self-insured plans offered to employees. Because employers were suspicious that HMOs attracted healthier employees, they resisted this requirement. The 1988 amendments provided greater flexibility in determining employer contributions to HMOs. (More detail concerning the 1988 amendments can be found in Chapter 5.)

## GROWTH OF DIFFERENT MODEL TYPES

During the early years of HMO development, the staff and group models tended to predominate. During the eighties, however, the IPAs became the dominant type of HMO. By the end of the decade, IPAs outnumbered all other plans by almost a two-to-one margin. While staff/group/network type HMOs had 81 percent of all HMO enrollees in 1980, they had only 57 percent in 1989. Nearly 400 IPAs in 1989 served 13.5 million members. Thus, from 1980 to 1989, the number of IPA plans increased approximately 300 percent, and IPA enrollment increased from 1.7 million to 13 million, an increase of almost 700 percent.

The IPAs grew rapidly for several reasons. First, physicians found IPAs the most acceptable form of HMO because they could join an IPA and still maintain the fee-for-service arrangement. Therefore, they often formed or joined IPAs in order to compete with other types of HMOs. Second, IPAs required significantly lower start-up costs, and therefore, financing could be more easily obtained for their development. Third, consumers often had a greater choice of providers in an IPA than in other types of HMOs. Indeed, many consumers who joined an IPA could retain the same physician they had before they signed.

## SIZE AND AGE OF HMOs

As can be seen in Table 2.2, at least three-fourths of all HMO enrollment is found in plans that have at least 50,000 members and over; half are in plans with at least 100,000 members. Likewise, over 60 percent of all HMO members are in plans at least ten years old. As small plans grow and as mergers among HMOs continue, a higher percentage of HMO enrollees belong to larger plans.

The decrease in small plans denotes the shift from small independent plans to larger, national HMO chains which started in the late seventies and accelerated in the eighties. (InterStudy defines a national HMO firm as having separate HMOs in two or more states.) In 1978, six national health firms had seventeen HMO plans that enrolled approximately half of all HMO members in the nation (3.7 million). By 1988, 41 national HMO firms had 320 affiliated HMOs that enrolled almost 18 million or nearly 60 percent of all HMO enrollment. Over half of these were enrolled in just four HMOs, each having more than one million enrollees. Although the Kaiser Foundation Health Plans still account for a large proportion of national HMO firm enrollment, it is evolving into the largest of several large firms rather than the giant among several much smaller firms (InterStudy, *National HMO Firms* 1988).

After a surge in 1985–1986, national HMO firms have maintained but have not increased their proportionate share of HMO firms. Multistate firms owned or managed 49 percent of all 653 HMOs operating in 1988. Similarly, the national firms' share of total HMO enrollment has remained about the same since 1985.

## REGIONAL DISTRIBUTION OF HMOs

While HMOs can be found across the nation, they tend to concentrate in certain areas of the country. HMOs' market penetration is greatest in the West and Southwest (California, Arizona, Utah, Colorado, Oregon, and Washington), in the upper Midwest (Minnesota, Wisconsin and Michigan), and in the Northeast (New York, Pennsylvania, New Jersey, and Connecticut) (See Table 2.3). Likewise, most of the HMO enrollment growth in recent years has been in the West and Northeast. HMOs have the lowest market share in the South and in the Midwest. Indeed, HMOs have lost enrollment in these two regions in recent years. The more conservative, independent orientations of both customers and providers in these regions may account for their lukewarm reception of HMOs.

California remains the state with the most HMO plans (sixty-one) and members (over eight million). Five states have over thirty HMOs (Florida, Illinois, New York, Ohio, and Texas) and ten states have more than one million members (Florida, Illinois, Massachusetts, Michigan, Minnesota, New York, Ohio, Pennsylvania, Texas, and Wisconsin).

**Table 2.2**
**January 1, 1990 Enrollment and Number of HMOs by Size, Age of Plan, Model Type, Federal Qualification Status, Profit Status, and Geographic Region**

| | PURE ENROLLMENT | | | | PLANS | | |
|---|---|---|---|---|---|---|---|
| | Total @ 1/1/90 | Percent of Total | Net Change 7/89-1/90 | Percent Change 7/89-1/90 | Total @ 1/1/90 | Percent of Total | Net Change 7/89-1/90 |
| **ALL PLANS** | **33,092,954** | **100.0** | **600,170** | **1.8** | **575** | **100.0** | **-15** |
| **Model Type:** | | | | | | | |
| Staff | 4,195,258 | 12.7 | 196,588 | 4.9 | 59 | 10.3 | -1 |
| Group | 9,317,170 | 28.2 | 139,687 | 1.5 | 65 | 11.3 | -1 |
| Network | 5,809,550 | 17.6 | 90,674 | 1.6 | 89 | 15.5 | -4 |
| IPA | 13,770,976 | 41.6 | 173,221 | 1.3 | 362 | 63.0 | -9 |
| **Size of Plan:*** | | | | | | | |
| 4,999 or less | 171,986 | .5 | -29,657 | -14.7 | 69 | 12.0 | -14 |
| 5,000 - 14,999 | 1,232,277 | 3.7 | 30,890 | 2.6 | 125 | 21.7 | -1 |
| 15,000 - 24,999 | 1,918,499 | 5.8 | -174,549 | -8.3 | 99 | 17.2 | -8 |
| 25,000 - 49,999 | 4,249,347 | 12.8 | 331,229 | 8.5 | 122 | 21.2 | 9 |
| 50,000 - 99,999 | 5,292,076 | 16.0 | -575,473 | -9.8 | 75 | 13.0 | -7 |
| 100,000 or more | 20,228,769 | 61.1 | 1,017,730 | 5.3 | 82 | 14.3 | 4 |
| **Age of Plan:** | | | | | | | |
| <1 year | 24,416 | .1 | -24,455 | -50.0 | 11 | 1.9 | -3 |
| 1-2 years | 869,717 | 2.6 | -610,720 | -41.0 | 71 | 12.3 | -45 |
| 3-5 years | 7,423,596 | 22.4 | 252,634 | 3.5 | 263 | 45.7 | 16 |
| 6-9 years | 4,811,930 | 14.5 | -155,044 | -3.1 | 86 | 15.0 | 6 |
| 10 or more | 19,963,295 | 60.3 | 1,137,755 | 6.0 | 144 | 25.0 | 11 |
| **Federal Qualification:** | | | | | | | |
| Qualified | 25,195,972 | 76.1 | 267,860 | 1.1 | 301 | 52.3 | -6 |
| Not Qualified | 7,896,982 | 23.9 | 332,310 | 4.4 | 274 | 47.7 | -9 |
| **Profit Status:** | | | | | | | |
| For-Profit | 15,166,079 | 45.8 | 162,829 | 1.1 | 377 | 65.6 | -16 |
| Not-For-Profit | 17,926,875 | 54.2 | 437,341 | 2.5 | 198 | 34.4 | 1 |
| **Geographic Region:** | | | | | | | |
| Northeast | 7,390,482 | 22.3 | 232,073 | 3.2 | 115 | 20.0 | -1 |
| South | 6,026,555 | 18.2 | 57,008 | 1.0 | 160 | 27.8 | -9 |
| Midwest | 7,591,208 | 22.9 | 63,499 | .8 | 176 | 30.6 | 1 |
| West | 12,019,701 | 36.3 | 240,919 | 2.0 | 121 | 21.0 | -6 |
| Guam | 65,008 | .2 | 6,671 | 11.4 | 3 | .5 | 0 |

*Three HMOs contain only open-ended enrollees and, as a result, are excluded from the Size of Plan Table.

*Source*: InterStudy, *The InterStudy Edge* (Excelsior, MN.: InterStudy, Spring, 1990). Reprinted with permission.

## FEDERAL QUALIFICATION

Following the 1973 HMO Act, many HMOs sought federal qualification in an effort to obtain grants and development funds from the federal government or to utilize the Act's provisions requiring employers to offer federally qualified

**Table 2.3**
**Pure State HMO Enrollment Ranked by Size of Enrollment: Percent of Population in HMOs—January 1, 1990**

| Ranking on 7/1/89 | State | Pure Enrollment | % of State Population in HMOs* |
|---|---|---|---|
| | **U.S. Total** | **33,092,954** | **13.3%** |
| 1 | 1. California | 8,693,538 | 29.9 |
| 2 | 2. New York | 2,646,416 | 14.7 |
| 3 | 3. Illinois | 1,501,523 | 12.9 |
| 4 | 4. Massachusetts | 1,482,798 | 25.1 |
| 5 | 5. Michigan | 1,421,657 | 15.3 |
| 7 | 6. Ohio | 1,353,359 | 12.4 |
| 8 | 7. Pennsylvania | 1,329,450 | 11.0 |
| 6 | 8. Florida | 1,319,655 | 10.4 |
| 9 | 9. Texas | 1,190,812 | 7.0 |
| 10 | 10. Wisconsin | 1,058,487 | 21.7 |
| 11 | 11. New Jersey | 901,375 | 11.7 |
| 13 | 12. Maryland | 747,136 | 15.9 |
| 12 | 13. Minnesota | 713,604 | 16.4 |
| 15 | 14. Washington | 678,883 | 14.3 |
| 14 | 15. Colorado | 661,039 | 19.9 |
| 16 | 16. Oregon | 657,016 | 23.3 |
| 17 | 17. Connecticut | 634,856 | 19.6 |
| 18 | 18. Arizona | 548,162 | 15.4 |
| 19 | 19. Missouri | 529,747 | 10.3 |
| 21 | 20. Indiana | 372,088 | 6.7 |
| 22 | 21. Virginia | 364,584 | 6.0 |
| 23 | 22. North Carolina | 309,073 | 4.7 |
| 29 | 23. Iowa | 300,398 | 10.6 |
| 24 | 24. Georgia | 297,603 | 4.6 |
| 25 | 25. Hawaii | 243,671 | 22.0 |
| 26 | 26. Louisiana | 235,751 | 5.4 |
| 28 | 27. Utah | 224,653 | 13.2 |
| 30 | 28. Rhode Island | 220,856 | 22.1 |
| 32 | 29. Kentucky | 217,848 | 5.8 |
| 31 | 30. Kansas | 217,609 | 8.7 |
| 34 | 31. Alabama | 212,207 | 5.2 |
| 27 | 32. Tennessee | 197,189 | 4.0 |
| 33 | 33. New Mexico | 193,800 | 12.7 |
| 35 | 34. Oklahoma | 162,748 | 5.0 |
| 37 | 35. New Hampshire | 111,308 | 10.1 |
| 36 | 36. Delaware | 111,605 | 14.8 |
| 38 | 37. Nevada | 91,709 | 8.3 |
| 39 | 38. Nebraska | 85,314 | 5.3 |
| 41 | 39. West Virginia | 70,766 | 3.8 |
| 40 | 40. South Carolina | 70,240 | 2.0 |
| 42 | 41. Arkansas | 50,495 | 2.1 |
| 45 | 42. Vermont | 33,128 | 5.8 |
| 46 | 43. Maine | 30,295 | 2.5 |
| 44 | 44. South Dakota | 26,522 | 3.7 |
| 48 | 45. Idaho | 23,820 | 2.3 |
| 47 | 46. North Dakota | 10,900 | 1.7 |
| 49 | 47. Montana | 3,410 | 0.4 |
| 20 | Dist. of Columbia | 468,843 | 77.6 |
| 43 | Guam | 65,008 | 49.6 |
| | Alaska | 0 | 0.0 |
| | Mississippi | 0 | 0.0 |
| | Wyoming | 0 | 0.0 |

*Source*: InterStudy, *The InterStudy Edge* (Excelsior, MN.: InterStudy, Spring 1990). Reprinted with permission.

*Note*: The District of Columbia has been excluded from the state ranking due to the significance of the cross-state nature of its enrollment. Guam has also been excluded from the ranking as it is not a state. However, both subjects remain in the totals.

*July 1, 1989 population estimates were provided by the U.S. Department of Commerce, Bureau of the Census.

HMO options to their employees. However, during the eighties, conditions encouraging HMOs to seek federal qualification began to change. In 1981, federal funding for the development of HMOs was phased out. As the HMO concept became much more familiar, and as employer resistance to HMOs decreased, the need for federal qualification to force an employer to accept an HMO also decreased. In addition, many HMOs wanted more flexibility than was allowed under federal qualification. Moreover, employers were less and less impressed with the quality assurances that were supposed to accompany federal qualification. While HMOs must initially have a quality assurance process to obtain federal qualification, there is little ongoing monitoring of the quality of health care delivery by the federal government in order to maintain qualification. Thus, many employers believe there are better ways to assure quality than too much reliance on federal qualification.

As a result of the above forces, the percentage of federally qualified HMOs has been declining in recent years. For example, in 1985, 63 percent of all HMOs were federally qualified, but by 1990, the percentage had dropped to 52 percent (see Table 2.2.). As HMOs scramble to offer more flexible options to employers in increasingly competitive markets, this trend toward noncertification and more flexibility will probably continue. On the other hand, one should remember that over 77 percent of HMO enrollees remain in federally qualified HMOs. It is still too early to tell if the 1988 amendments to the HMO Act, which eased federal requirements for qualification, will encourage significantly more HMOs to seek federal qualification.

## PROFIT VERSUS NONPROFIT

In the 1970s, most HMOs were nonprofit. However, in 1983, financial analysts gave favored status to the HMO industry (Gruber et al. 1988). As a result, many HMOs, hungry for capital, converted from nonprofit to for-profit organizations. Most of the new IPA-model HMOs, which have had the fastest growth in recent years, have been for-profit. With the exception of the Kaiser plans, for-profit HMOs tend to dominate the industry today.

## BENEFIT TRENDS IN HMOs

Table 2.4 summarizes the extent to which various benefits were covered in HMOs' best-selling benefit packages in 1988 (Gold and Hodges 1989). While specific benefits are negotiated between employers and HMOs, there is much consistency among the benefit plans provided different groups. Approximately 68 percent of plan enrollees were covered under the best-selling package. Regardless of qualification status, essentially all HMOs provided benefits that are required of federally qualified HMOs (Gold and Hodges 1989). These included primary care, outpatient lab and x ray, hospitalization, emergency, prenatal and home health care, outpatient care, and physical therapy. Over 90 percent of the

**Table 2.4**
**Overview of Coverage of Selected Benefits in Health Maintenance Organization Plans Over Three Years Old, 1988[a]**

| Virtually always covered (99 percent or more of plans) | |
|---|---|
| Primary care visits (100 percent)[b] | Typically no limits; half charge copayments |
| Outpatient laboratory (100 percent)[b] | Typically no limits or copayments (13 percent have copayments) |
| Outpatient x-ray (100 percent)[b] | Typically no limits or copayments (14 percent have copayments) |
| Prenatal care (100 percent)[b] | Typically no limits; one-third charge copayments |
| Emergency care (100 percent)[b] | Typically no limits; two-thirds charge copayments |
| Hospitalization (99 percent)[b] | Typically no limits or copayments (14 percent have copayments) |
| Home health care (100 percent)[b] | Two-thirds have no limits or copayments; the rest vary |
| Outpatient mental health care (100 percent)[b] | Typically with limits and copayments (21 percent have limits only) |
| Physical therapy (100 percent)[b] | No clear pattern on benefit structures (61 percent have limits) |
| **Almost always covered (90–98 percent of plans)** | |
| Allergy treatment (98 percent) | Typically no limits or copayments, or copayments only |
| Drug/alcohol detoxification (98 percent)[b] | No clear pattern; 56 percent have limits and one-third copayments |
| Skilled nursing care (97 percent) | Over half of plans have limits; copayments are rarer |
| Inhalation therapy (96 percent)[b] | Half have no limits or copayments; the rest vary but copayments are common |
| Pharmacy (94 percent) | Usually with copayments; sometimes with limits |
| Hearing tests (94 percent)[b] | Half have no limits or copayments; copayments more common than limits |
| Speech therapy (92 percent)[b] | Usually with limits; sometimes with copayments |
| Vision tests (91 percent)[b] | No clear pattern on benefit structure; copayments more common than limits |
| Inpatient mental health care (91 percent) | Almost always with limits; sometimes with copayments |
| **Usually covered (65–89 percent of plans)** | |
| Dental/accidental injury (86 percent) | Two-fifths cover without limits or copayments; others vary |
| Occupational therapy (85 percent)[b] | No clear pattern on benefit structure; over half have limits |
| Drug/alcohol rehabilitation (81 percent) | Usually with limits, with or without copayments |
| Hospice (80 percent) | Typically with no limits or copayments, or just limits |
| External prosthetics (77 percent) | No clear pattern on benefit structure |
| Podiatry (78 percent) | Half covering have no limits or copayments; copayments common in rest |
| Durable medical equipment (76 percent) | No clear pattern on benefit structure |
| **Sometimes covered (25–64 percent of plans)** | |
| Chiropractic services (45 percent) | Half cover with no limits or copayments; the rest vary |
| Temporomandibular joint treatment (43 percent) | No clear pattern on benefit structure |
| **Least frequently covered (0–24 percent of plans)** | |
| Preventive dental care (23 percent) | No clear pattern on benefit structure |
| Eyeglasses (18 percent) | Typically with limits, with or without copayments |
| In vitro fertilization (17 percent) | No clear pattern or benefit structure |
| Restorative dental care (13 percent) | No clear pattern on benefit structure |
| Hearing aids (12 percent) | Typically with limits |
| Cosmetic surgery (7 percent) | Typically with limits; copayments are rarer |

*Source*: GHAA Annual HMO Industry Survey, 1988. As summarized in M. Gold and D. Hodges. *Health Affairs* 8 (1989): p. 127. Reprinted with permission.

[a]Based on best-selling benefit package (excluding Medicare or Medicaid) including riders typically purchased with package. Descriptions of benefits are based on responses indicating whether or not the amount of service or dollar expenditure is restricted, and whether or not any patient cost-sharing is required

[b]Required coverage for federally qualified plans under the HMO Act. Vision and hearing tests are only required for children through age seventeen.

unprofitable HMOs became even more unprofitable in 1985 (InterStudy, *Bottom Line* 1989). Profits declined even more in 1986.

A Group Health Association of America (GHAA) survey revealed that only 40 percent of the responding HMOs realized a profit in 1986 (*Financial Performance* 1988). Moreover, some large HMOs and HMO chains had losses at year end. In 1987, the losses continued to grow as over 70 percent of all HMOs reported pretax losses. Thus, while enrollments increased dramatically in 1985, 1986, and 1987, profits fell. Apparently, HMOs were placing emphasis on growth and market share at the expense of profitability (InterStudy, *Bottom Line* 1989).

While HMOs increased premiums during 1985–1987, the increases trailed well behind the 20 percent to 50 percent premium increases of indemnity plans. HMOs increased premiums just under 3 percent between 1985 and 1986 and just over 7 percent between 1986 and 1987. From January 1987 to January 1988, premium increases were just under 12 percent (InterStudy, *Bottom Line* 1989). These premium increases also trailed employee health benefit costs as noted in the Foster Higgins annual health care benefits surveys. In 1986, the costs per employee increased 7.7 percent (Johnson and Higgins, 1986). Similarly, costs increased 7.9 percent in 1987 (Foster Higgins 1987). In 1988, costs escalated dramatically averaging 8.6 percent higher than in 1987 (Foster Higgins 1988). Thus, while HMO premiums were increasing approximately 22 percent from 1985 through 1987, employee health care costs were escalating over 34 percent. Sacrificing financial stability for growth, and market penetration for profits could not be sustained for long. Likewise, the premiums of new members could offset losses for only awhile. As a result, forty-two HMOs failed during 1988.

The Maxicare Plans were the most notable failure. Maxicare grew out of a California HMO and became the largest national HMO (in terms of number of plans) in 1986 when it acquired two other HMO firms. Maxicare paid over $445 million for the two firms which more than doubled its enrollment to over two million members in thirty-seven HMOs in twenty-five states (*InterStudy Edge* Spring 1989).

Maxicare sought to become a national system of health care by developing a national accounts program for multistate employers which provided standardized benefit packages, enrollment procedures and single billings separated by location (*InterStudy Edge* Spring 1989). However, Maxicare may have selected the worst time to become a national giant. Tough competition from other HMOs and the new PPOs provided no relief for Maxicare. The company struggled in 1987, and its difficulties were exacerbated by the stock market decline of October 1987. By January 1, 1989, Maxicare owned only sixteen HMOs in thirteen states. It closed another seven plans during the first few months of 1989. Finally, March 15, 1989, Maxicare filed for Chapter 11 bankruptcy.

Maxicare's fall provides a lesson for the management of HMOs. Health care remains a local and regional effort. Physician practice patterns and approaches differ greatly among locales and from region to region. Contracting practices between physicians and HMOs also differ. Likewise, employer desires and ex-

**Table 2.5**
**Average of Preventive Services in Best-Selling Benefit Package, 1988**

| Type of Benefit | Percent Offered in Best-Selling Package |
|---|---|
| Well Baby Care | 100 |
| Pap Smears | 100 |
| Mammography—Diagnostic | 100 |
| Mammography—Screening | 99 |
| Influenza Shots | 98 |
| Child Immunization | 99 |
| Adult Immunization | 97 |
| Routine Physical | 99 |
| School/Work Physical | 35 |
| Nutrition Counseling | 85 |
| Health Education Classes | 76 |

*Source*: GHAA Annual HMO Industry Survey, 1988

plans covered allergy treatment, drug and alcohol detoxification, skilled nursing care, pharmacy benefits, hearing and vision tests, speech therapy, and inpatient mental health care.

In addition to the preventive/wellness services noted in Table 2.4 (primary care, prenatal care, speech and hearing tests), HMOs offered the services noted in Table 2.5. The copayment for the services in Table 2.5 generally ranged between 20 and 30 percent. The extensive first dollar coverage by most HMOs combined with HMOs' emphasis on preventive services often attracted families and women in the childbearing years (Gold and Hodges 1989). These groups tended to be disproportionately represented in HMOs.

In recent years, there has been more interest in HMOs' mental health and substance abuse services. While nearly all plans provided these benefits, limits, and copayments were imposed on the use of them. In mental health services, twenty outpatient visits and thirty inpatient days were common limits. Nearly 80 percent required some payment for outpatient mental health services which averaged $16 per visit in 1988. Approximately one-third of the plans required payment for inpatient mental health services. In substance abuse services, limits, and copayments were less common for detoxification services than for rehabilitation services (Gold and Hodges 1989).

## FINANCIAL HEALTH OF HMOs

Although HMO enrollments were surging in 1985 through 1987, profits were not. Overall net income per member declined in profitable HMOs, and the pectations differ from market to market (*InterStudy Edge* Spring 1989). Maxicare may have sought to centralize too much out of Los Angeles. Other national firms also experienced losses in 1987. Humana lost over $66 million; Lincoln National lost over $50 million; United Health Care lost over $16 million; and Equicor and CIGNA absorbed substantial losses.

With the collapse of Maxicare and the troubles of other HMOs, states became more concerned about the financial solvency of HMOs and called for stricter HMO financial reserve requirements. At the same time, it became more difficult for HMOs, particularly new ones, to find capital.

In 1988, only 36 percent of HMO plans responding to an InterStudy Survey reported a net profit (InterStudy, *Bottom Line* 1989). The unprofitable HMOs indicated three major reasons for losses: (1) higher outpatient costs, (2) higher outpatient utilization, and (3) higher inpatient costs. Other significant reasons were higher inpatient utilization and higher administrative costs.

Younger HMO plans tended to be the least profitable. In 1988, only 20 percent of those HMOs in operation for three years or less were profitable. Young HMOs had less available cash to meet state regulations. They would sometimes stretch out payments to vendors and providers in order to conserve cash (Marion Digest 1989). Although young HMOs' reserves climbed 42 percent in 1988, expenses climbed faster, and most ended the year with losses almost double those of 1987.

After comparing the profitability of different HMO models, it is clear the IPAs were the least profitable. Only one-fourth of the IPAs reported a profit. In contrast, over half of staff and network models reported a profit in 1988. Hence, it is not surprising that staff and network models had the lowest median costs per member in 1988 for both physician services and inpatient hospital care. Moreover, staff models had the best liquidity in 1988. Also, nonprofit and federally funded HMOs tended to have more profits.

Within the last two years, the financial outlook for HMOs has improved with more HMOs reporting profits. High premiums are the most obvious reason for this improved financial condition. Premium increases of 20 to 30 percent were common in 1989 (InterStudy, *National Managed Care Firms* 1989). Other reasons include improved utilization controls, more favorable provider contracts, better control of administrative contracts and dropping of unprofitable groups from the HMO.

## TRENDS IN HMO PREMIUMS AND COPAYMENTS

HMO premiums in 1988 were almost 12 percent higher than in 1987, and in 1989, they were over 16 percent higher than in 1988. Likewise, rates in 1990 were approximately 16 percent higher than in 1989. Although these increases were above the consumer price index, they were still several points below the average increases for regular indemnity plans. The increases were lowest for group and staff-model plans and for older, larger and nonprofit HMOs. Also, the HMOs which were profitable in 1988 tended to have lower premium increases than those that did not report a profit.

Copayment increases became more frequent in 1989 when almost 40 percent of HMOs reported increasing a copayment. Copayment increases were most common for prescription drugs followed by increased copayments for physician office and emergency room visits. Copayments were highest for emergency room visits and mental health services. Among the various types of HMOs, staff models tended to have the lowest copayments.

## COMPETITION AND HMOs

During the last several years, HMOs have faced intense competition from other managed care organizations such as preferred provider organizations (PPOs). As a result, many HMOs have seen their enrollment growth decline in 1988 and 1989. At the same time, employers have been pressuring HMOs to provide more flexibility in their options. As a result, new HMO hybrid products have developed such as "open-ended HMOs" and "triple-option plans."

Open-ended HMOs allow the enrollee to use non-HMO providers without referrals when the enrollee pays a higher fee generally in the form of a deductible and coinsurance. While open-ended enrollments are less than 20 percent of all HMO enrollments, they are increasing at a much faster rate than overall HMO enrollments. The chief attraction of the open-ended option is the greater selection of providers it allows.

Triple-option plans provide the HMO option, a preferred provider option, and a traditional indemnity insurance. These plans provide consumers the choice of health care from an HMO with no out-of-pocket expense, or nonplan HMO physicians through the PPO, or through the traditional insurance when deductible and coinsurance are paid. Thus, the enrollees can decide at the point of service which plan they wish to use. Approximately half of all national HMO firms now offer multiple options, and the other half offer PPOs and other managed care products outside the regular HMOs, such as dental HMOs, mental health HMOs, utilization review services, and so on.

Employers have also pressed for more experience-based ratings or premiums. Traditionally, HMOs have used community ratings (average health care costs of all employees in the HMO) to determine the premiums charged an employer. However, as employers have become more concerned that their healthier employees are attracted to HMOs, they have pressed HMOs to provide more data on the actual costs of health care for their particular employees, and have urged HMOs to base their companies' premiums on the actual experience of their employees. For the first time, the HMO Act Amendments of 1988 allowed federally qualified HMOs to adjust rates prospectively for the experience of employer groups. Over 30 percent of all plans expect to use experience ratings in the future (Gold and Hodges 1989).

## THE FUTURE OF HMOs

As a result of pressure from employers, HMOs will continue to experiment with hybrid options. Likewise, traditional indemnity insurance companies will offer products that often look very similar to HMOs but are not called or licensed as HMOs. Thus, we will see a continuing blurring of lines among traditional options. However, one of the greatest selling points for HMOs is the comprehensive benefits and low out-of-pocket costs. If HMOs move too far away from this concept, they will lose much of their appeal (Gold and Hodges 1989). HMOs must learn which products they can manage well and which are adaptable to the traditional HMO features.

Finally, as HMOs' premiums increase and as employers become much more concerned about the true savings and quality provided by HMOs, successful HMOs will become much more proficient at gathering, analyzing, and displaying specific data to employers which document both quality and cost effectiveness.

The big shake out of the HMO industry is probably over. Growth in HMOs will be stable, but not spectacular. Emphasis will probably shift from growth in enrollment to greater concerns about providing and measuring quality, more aggressive efforts to influence physician practice styles, and greater attention to cost-containment strategies for outpatient and ambulatory services (Gruber et al. 1988).

# 3

# Utilization and Costs in HMOs

While there are several reasons for the development of HMOs, chief among them is the desire to control costs. HMOs are structured so that, at least in theory, they have both the incentive and capacity to reduce the growth in health care expenditures. Since HMOs seem to be effective in reducing utilization, particularly hospitalization, they are able to reduce costs. But are these reductions maintained across time? Are they cumulative, or is there only a one-time reduction? These are some of the questions that need to be addressed.

In addition to decreasing utilization and thereby controlling costs, HMOs could also reduce expenditures by improving the efficiency of their operations. But some critics of HMOs contend that they do not cut costs at all, and that they are not more efficient. Rather, the critics say, HMOs attract low-risk, lower-cost individuals into their plans, so that they only appear to cut costs because they have a comparatively healthy population. This issue of "biased selection" is discussed in considerable detail as are the techniques that HMOs might employ to encourage enrollment of low-risk individuals. Finally, the strategies that employers can use to discourage such favorable selection are outlined.

## DIFFERENT APPROACHES TO MEDICAL PRACTICE AND UTILIZATION

There are numerous economic and noneconomic variables that suggest utilization and thus costs of medical care in HMOs will be lower than in the Fee-For-Service (FFS) system. Table 3.1 provides a summary of these variables for three major systems of health delivery, (1) the conventional FFS system and insurance, (2) the individual practice association (IPA) type of HMO, and

**Table 3.1**
**Probable Effects on Utilization of Services of Various Factors in Different Practice Settings**

| Type of Medical Care/ Rationing Factors | Conventional Fee-for-Service and Insurance | |
|---|---|---|
| Patient Initiated Visits | | |
| Price to consumer | Initial and preventive visits often not covered | - |
| Knowledge of provider | Often a local physician with a long standing relationship | + |
| Appointment lag | Typically short, urgent visits "squeezed in" | + |
| Accessibility to provider | Decentralized, likely one close to patient | + |
| Waiting time in office | Variable, often long because patients "squeezed in" | - |
| Physician Initiated Visits | | |
| Physician incentives | Follow-up increases revenue | + |
| Other factors similar to above | | |
| Physician Initiated Referral | | |
| Physician incentives | Reciprocal referrals among different specialists encouraged by professional network, discouraged by prohibitions on fee splitting | + |
| Price to consumer | More likely covered than initial visit, still not complete | +/- |
| Accessibility to provider | Typically at different location | - |
| Incentives to "return patients to primary care physician" | Depends on nature of referral network | + |
| Hospitalization | | |
| Price to patient | Often fairly comprehensive coverage but some payments | - |
| Incentives for physician | Hourly income higher in hospital | + |

+ = tends to increase utilization
- = tends to decrease utilization
+/- = mixed effects

(3) the prepaid group practice plan (PGP) type of HMO (Group, Network, and Staff-Model HMOs).

## Selection of Physician

In the FFS system, the consumer does not behave as a typical customer in nonhealth care markets. Compared with consumers of other products, patients often have much less information about medical practice, medical outcomes, and costs. As a result, the patient often does not know who is providing the

**Table 3.1 (continued)**

| IPA-HMOs: Fee-for-Service Practitioners at Risk | | PGP-HMOs | |
|---|---|---|---|
| Comprehensive coverage of all visits | + | Comprehensive coverage of all visits | + |
| Often a local physician with a longstanding relationship | + | Often a local physician with no prior contact with patient | - |
| Typically short, urgent visits "squeezed in" | + | Typically long, urgent visits routed to separate clinic | - |
| Decentralized, likely one close to patient | + | Centralized, generally further from patient | - |
| Variable, often long because patients "squeezed in" | - | Typically short if appointment made in advance | + |
| Follow-up increases revenue more than risk sharing | + | Follow-up reduces net income; substitute call backs | - |
| Referrals encouraged by professional network but discouraged by risk sharing | +/- | Referral attractive to "dump" a problem patient but collegial and financial costs if frequent | - |
| Comprehensive coverage of all visits | + | Comprehensive coverage of all visits | + |
| Typically at a different location | - | Centralized--"one stop care" | + |
| Depends on referral network, sometimes encouraged by HMO | +/- | Typically encouraged by the system | - |
| Comprehensive coverage pays in full | + | Comprehensive coverage pays in full | + |
| Hourly income higher but risk sharing tends to counter | +/- | No additional income, costs are borne by plan | - |

*Source*: H. S. Luft. "Health Maintenance Organizations and the Rationing of Medical Care." *Health and Society* 60 (1982): 276 and 277. Reprinted with permission.

most cost-effective medical care. Thus, the patient may lack sufficient information to select the most cost-effective physician.

Since patients are generally sick or injured when seeking a physician, their immediate concern is to find a doctor who can properly diagnose and treat their problem. The price and utilization of the care is not the primary concern when illness or injury is acute. Combined with other factors in the FFS system, this customer or patient ignorance tends to encourage utilization.

In HMOs, the patient or customer selects an HMO option that provides a set of benefits together with a price. The selection of HMO coverage is thus made long in advance of illness or injury. Thus, individuals are more able and likely to select a more cost-effective plan than could occur when there is an immediate and more pressing need to locate a physician.

### Price to Consumer

Under the FFS system, the initial and preventive visits to a physician often are not covered because the deductible must first be paid before insurance is available. Thus, the deductible tends to decrease utilization.

In both IPA and PGP model HMOs, comprehensive coverage without deductible is provided. Likewise, preventive visits are often paid in full. These arrangements in HMOs tend to increase utilization.

### Knowledge of Provider

Under the FFS system, the patient often goes to a local physician with whom the patient has generally had a long-standing relationship. The fact that the patient is familiar with his or her doctor encourages greater utilization.

Patients in IPAs often have long-standing relationships with their physicians which in turn increase utilization. However, in many PGPs, patients may go to a doctor who they have not previously seen. The lack of a long-standing relationship tends to discourage utilization.

### Appointment Day

Patients in the FFS system typically can arrange an office visit in a relatively short period of time. Similarly, if it is an urgent visit, they can generally be "squeezed in" the doctor's schedule. Basically, the same can occur in an IPA. Therefore, ease of appointments encourages utilization in both FFS and IPA arrangements.

Appointments typically take longer in PGPs and urgent visits may be sent to a separate clinic. Because of this time lag in getting an appointment, utilization is discouraged in PGPs.

### Accessibility to Provider

In the FFS system, patients generally live near a primary care physician. Likewise, the IPA general practitioner is often nearby. This accessibility encourages utilization. PGP physicians, however, may not be relatively close and greater travel time may be required. Logically, this tends to discourage utilization.

If the FFS or IPA primary care physician recommends a specialist, the patient will probably have to travel to a separate location which could discourage utilization. On the other hand, the PGP specialist may be in the same centralized location as the primary care physician. This proximity encourages utilization in the PGP.

### Waiting Time in Office

The waiting time in primary care physician offices may be long because more urgent patients are often "squeezed in" under the FFS and IPA arrangements. This wait tends to discourage utilization. In contrast, the waiting time in a PGP office tends to be short if an appointment is arranged. As a result, utilization tends to increase.

### Physician Incentives

In the FFS system, the physician is paid for the number and kind of services provided. Likewise, the primary care physician acts as the agent for the patient and decides if other medical services such as tests, hospitalization, or other medical specialists are needed. All of these providers are typically paid on a fee-for-service or cost-reimbursement basis by the patient's insurer. Thus, since neither the patient nor the provider must absorb most of the costs, the amount of medical care provided is likely to increase.

In the IPA, the participating physicians receive discounted fees for their services. While an individual physician could earn more money by providing more services, he could lose money if the physicians collectively in the IPA order too much or too expensive services. Therefore, the IPA physician is subject to conflicting pressures. The IPA physician's incentive to do more may be only partially offset by the collective risk-sharing. This may be particularly true in IPAs where the IPA patients account for under 15 percent of the physicians' caseload (Luft 1982; Meier and Tillotson 1978).

Physician incentives within PGPs would appear to discourage utilization. Since an annual capitation fee for each patient is paid to the HMO rather than fees for each service delivered, PGP physicians have an economic incentive to provide fewer services. In PGPs, physicians are generally paid by salaries and bonuses or by a fee-for-service based system modified to reflect the total pool of funds available. The salary system tends to discourage greater utilization because the physician is paid the same salary regardless of the number of services provided. Indeed, overutilization could endanger the physician's salary increase or bonus.

### Malpractice Threats

In the FFS system, physicians may err on the side of more medical care and more tests in order to protect themselves against malpractice suits. As a result, utilization is encouraged. The same probably holds in the IPA where the patient might sue both the doctor and the HMO. However, in the PGP where the doctor is employed by the HMO and where the HMO purchases malpractice insurance and is likely to be the object of a suit, the physician may be less concerned about the threat of malpractice suits. Thus, PGP physicians may be more conservative when prescribing tests and procedures. As a result, utilization may decrease.

### Hospitalization

In the FFS system, there is generally comprehensive coverage for hospitalization, but there are some copayments. These tend to discourage hospitalization. On the other hand, since HMOs generally have comprehensive coverage without copayments, hospitalization would be encouraged. However, the doctor, not the patient, generally determines when and how long a patient is hospitalized. Physicians under conventional fee-for-service have an incentive to hospitalize in that their hourly income tends to be higher in the hospital.

In the IPA arrangement, the doctor's hourly income would increase in the hospital, but hospitalization of the patient also would reduce the collective pool of the IPA physicians. These two conflicting trends would tend to balance.

In a PGP, the doctor receives no more income if the patient is hospitalized. Indeed, hospitalization would drive up the total HMO costs and thus endanger potential physician bonuses. Hence, the PGP physician would be less likely to suggest hospitalization of a patient.

### Summary of Factors Affecting Utilization

From the above discussion and Table 3.1, we can predict that hospital utilization will be highest in the FFS system, less in an IPA arrangement and least in a PGP. Likewise, the use of specialists would appear to be higher in the FFS system, lower in an IPA and lowest in the PGP.

On the other hand, the initial use of primary care physicians may be higher among PGP and lower in the IPA and FFS arrangements. However, the comprehensive coverage of both types of HMOs combined with the plans' efforts to discourage costly hospitalization may encourage more ambulatory care in both types of HMOs as compared to the FFS system.

## UTILIZATION

The discussion above considers the theoretical factors that are predicted to influence utilization. The following section reviews various empirical studies of utilization to see if the predictions are correct. The two primary areas of health care utilization are hospital and ambulatory care.

### Hospital Utilization

HMOs are more interested in controlling hospitalization than physician visits or other ambulatory care. It is difficult for HMOs to monitor and control physician visits because of the great number and because they are initiated by patients. On the other hand, nearly all hospitalizations are initiated by physicians. As a result, HMOs hope to achieve lower hospitalization through their physicians and the internal policies of the HMO. Moreover, hospital costs tend to be much higher than ambulatory care. When given a choice, HMOs will choose less costly ambulatory care over hospitalization. Hence, HMOs will concentrate on what is most costly and most controllable.

Luft (1981) reviewed twenty-six studies that included fifty-seven comparisons of hospital utilization among HMOs and other providers. He compared the number of inpatient days per 1,000 enrollees or 1,000 member years. Total inpatient days are the product of total admissions per enrollee times the average length of stay per admission (Luft 1981). In forty-three of the fifty-seven pairs, HMO enrollees had fewer hospital days than the comparison group, and in forty-six, the admission rate was lower. HMOs in Luft's study averaged 20 to 40 percent lower admission rates than comparison FFS groups. PGPs had notably lower admission rates than IPAs.

One major criticism of the studies reviewed by Luft was that they did not contain controlled trials that randomly assigned patients to HMOs and FFS arrangements and which held most other variables constant. After Luft's study, the Rand Health Insurance Experiment provided such a controlled trial. Some 1,580 patients were randomly assigned to receive care free of charge from either a fee-for-service physician of their choice or the Group Health Cooperative of Puget Sound (a PGP type HMO). The rate of hospital admissions in the HMO was 40 percent lower than those in the fee-for-service group. These reductions under controlled conditions parallel those noted by Luft's review.

More recent data from the Health Care Financing Administration reveal that among medicare enrollees, HMOs achieved a 19 percent reduction in hospital admissions (Langwell et al. 1987). Similar results were found by Nelson, Rossiter, and Adamache (1986) in their study of medicare enrollees in HMOs.

As a result of these studies, we can safely say that HMOs do reduce hospital admissions and that PGPs are more effective in reducing admissions than IPAs.

Hospital admissions and length of stay combine to determine the total number of inpatient days. HMOs do not appear to be as effective in limiting the length of stay in hospitals. This may result from the conflicting objectives in HMOs. On the one hand, HMOs have economic incentives to limit stays in hospitals to a minimum. Yet, on the other hand, HMOs seek to keep hospital admissions to a minimum. To the extent that HMOs successfully reduce admissions, they keep the less serious cases out of the hospital. As a result, HMOs tend to have more serious patients admitted to the hospital who in turn will have longer stays.

Some critics of HMOs say that lower hospital utilization within HMOs results at least in part from unreported medical care received by HMO enrollees through out-of-plan utilization. These critics say that HMO rates reflect only the hospital admissions that the HMOs know about and pay for, not the total hospital experience of their enrollees. This can occur when another insurer or institution pays (e.g., Medicare, No Fault, Workmen's Compensation, duplicate coverage by a spouse, school health and liability insurance, VA or military insurance), or when the HMO does not cover the procedure (e.g., cosmetic or oral surgery, long-term psychiatric or rehabilitation stays), or when HMO coverage is denied for procedural reasons (Mott 1986). However, research indicates that out-of-plan utilization is not a major problem since the data suggest that such usage is low and ranges from 1 percent (Gaus, Kooper, and Hirschman 1976) to about 8 percent (Columbia University 1962).

As traditional insurers in the fee-for-service sector become more proficient in managed care (i.e., preadmission certification, second opinions, concurrent review, case management), the capacity of HMOs to reduce admissions will be reduced. In other words, many of the controls long utilized by HMOs are being adopted by traditional insurers. Thus, HMOs will have a less inflated number of hospital admissions in the fee-for-service sector to reduce, and as a result, HMOs' savings may not appear as dramatic as they have in the past.

### Ambulatory Care

While it appears clear that HMOs can reduce hospital utilization, their capacity to reduce outpatient care is much less apparent. Unlike hospital care, where HMOs have strong incentives to reduce utilization, the incentives concerning ambulatory care are mixed. HMOs have incentives to substitute ambulatory care for more expensive hospital care. Likewise, HMOs may encourage more preventive visits to physicians in order to avoid more serious and costly hospital care. On the other hand, the capitation system of HMOs discourages all utilization both outpatient and inpatient.

HMO enrollees have an incentive to use more ambulatory care because one capitation payment pays for all services used. Thus, the number of patient-initiated visits should be higher in HMOs. However, follow-up visits are scheduled by the HMO physician whose incentives would seem to discourage follow-ups.

It is more difficult to compare ambulatory care among HMOs and FFS providers because it is difficult to define an ambulatory visit. Do only physician visits count or do visits to allied health professionals also count? Is a visit to a physician followed by several tests, x rays, and procedures administered by others in the same building constitute only one or several visits?

Despite these methodological problems, a number of studies have compared ambulatory use in HMOs with that of FFS groups. Luft (1981) reviewed twenty-nine such studies and found that in nineteen of the comparisons, HMO enrollees had a larger number of patient-initiated visits. IPAs were particularly likely to have such visits. On the other hand, the physician-initiated follow-up visits did not show a clear pattern. The Rand experiment revealed no significant differences in outpatient visits among HMOs and FFS groups (Manning et al. 1984). A more recent review of ambulatory use studies by Hulka and Wheat (1985) indicates that HMOs tend to encourage more patient-initiated and prevention visits but discourage follow-up and illness visits. From these studies, there appears to be a small tendency for HMOs, particularly IPAs, to encourage more patient-initiated ambulatory visits and a small tendency for HMOs, particularly PGPs, to discourage follow-up and referral visits.

## COSTS IN HMOs VERSUS FFS

Most reviews of cost comparisons between HMOs and FFS plans reveal that the total cost of medical care (premiums plus out-of-pocket expenses) are lower for HMO enrollees than for comparable persons covered by conventional insurance plans. This difference ranges from 10 to 40 percent depending on the characteristics of the HMO. The greatest savings have been reported in California's Kaiser-Permanente plans which have averaged 50 percent lower costs per enrollee than costs in Blue Cross/Blue Shield (Luft 1978).

Data from the controlled experiment sponsored by the Rand Corporation indicate that HMOs can reduce costs by approximately 25 percent (Manning et al. 1984). Most of these savings came from reduced hospitalization in HMOs. Likewise, Welch, Frank, and Diehr (1984) found that the costs of a PGP were at least 33 percent lower than costs for a conventional insurer. As with utilization, costs vary considerably among the different types of HMOs. IPAs tend to have the highest costs of any HMO, while PGPs tend to have the lowest.

## TRENDS IN HMO COSTS VERSUS FFS COSTS

While it is clear that the cost of care in HMOs at any point in time is lower than FFS costs, is this reduction a one-time reduction or do HMOs have a lower rate of cost increases over time? If HMOs can provide only a one-time cost reduction, their capacity to control national health care costs is considerably limited. In other words, growth of HMOs would temporarily reduce the rate of growth, but once the portion of the population enrolled in HMOs leveled off, then the old rate of increase would resume. Luft's review of federal employees in HMOs and conventional insurance plans between 1961 and 1974 reveals that HMOs experienced slightly lower rates of growth (Luft 1981). PGP enrollees had annual premium increases of 1 to 1.5 percentage points lower than those in conventional insurance plans, while IPA enrollees had increases of 3.6 points lower.

A subsequent review of cost trends in 45 HMOs by Newhouse et al. (1985) indicates that the cost increases for HMOs and conventional plans were very similar. The authors concluded that over a two decade period the rate of HMO cost increases was the same as in the FFS system. These studies tend to indicate that HMOs' costs rise at the same or slightly lower rates than do those in the traditional FFS system. Thus, HMOs appear to achieve a one-time reduction in costs. While they maintain this reduction across time, they increase it very little if at all over time.

## EFFICIENCY IN HMOs

As we have seen, much of the cost savings produced by HMOs results from their lower levels of utilization, particularly hospitalization. It is possible that some cost reductions could result from greater efficiency within HMOs. In other words, HMOs may be able to produce a unit of health care (e.g., physician visit, costs per hospital admission) more efficiently than FFS providers. Since HMOs know the number and mix of populations they serve, it is theoretically possible that they may be better able to match facilities and personnel with that population and reduce excess or underutilized resources.

Since most HMOs do not own their own hospitals, it is difficult for the HMOs to achieve greater efficiencies in hospitals. Moreover, most HMOs contract with hospitals in which the HMO admissions may constitute only a small minority of all admissions. Therefore, the impact of HMOs on a hospital's operations is limited. Yet, Johnson and Aquilina (1986) found that HMO hospital resource use in the Minneapolis/St. Paul area as measured by length-of-stay was lower than for other payers even after controlling for the length-of-stay effects of case-mix differences.

In HMO-owned or controlled hospitals, Luft (1981) found that there was 5 to 28 percent lower costs per case. This efficiency is often achieved by using fewer personnel who are often more highly paid than similar personnel in non-HMO hospitals. When HMOs own their hospitals, they also tend to avoid duplication of facilities. Community hospitals, however, may purchase specialized, latest technology equipment in order to compete for physicians and their patients. Often such equipment is not fully utilized. HMO-controlled hospitals do not face this problem. HMOs which own hospitals tend to centralize certain types of care in different hospitals so that each hospital does not compete with others. Laboratory facilities also tend to be centralized so that there are fewer slack resources.

It is very difficult to study efficiency in the delivery of ambulatory services because it is difficult to define a unit of service. What constitutes a patient visit? Moreover, not all visits are alike. Recognizing these limitations, most evidence indicates that when the effects of group practice are held constant, an HMO has little additional impact on productivity and efficiency.

There appears to be only a small economy of scale in physicians' medical practices. While group practice appears to be more efficient than solo practice, maximum productivity or lowest cost per visit appears to occur when there are two to four physicians. Beyond four, physician productivity tends to fall and expenses per physician tend to increase (Luft 1981). This relationship holds whether the group is in an HMO or in a traditional FFS arrangement. Thus, the existence of an HMO seems to have little impact beyond the effects of group practice on economies or efficiency in the delivery of outpatient care.

## HMOs' IMPACT ON NON-HMO COSTS

As we have already seen, HMOs operate on a fixed budget for a given number of enrollees and have internal economic incentives to manage patient care efficiently and to reduce utilization. Hence, they are particularly adept at reducing inpatient utilization. As a result, the price offered by HMOs for a given level of benefits is generally lower than that offered by FFS providers. Competition advocates like Walter McClure (1978) and Alain Enthoven (1980) have contended that as HMOs increase their total enrollment and achieve greater efficiency primarily by lowering hospital utilization, by using fewer resources once a patient is admitted, and by controlling significant amounts of patient volume, they become strong price competitors with hospitals. As a result, non-HMO hospitals, physicians and insurers will strive to match HMO performance. Thus, as HMOs gain large market shares, the combined pressures of HMOs will require hospitals and other third-party buyers to become more price conscious and cost effective (Feldman et al. 1986).

The results of research on the competitive impact of HMOs on non-HMO providers is mixed. Chiswick (1976) conducted an analysis of the variation in occupancy and admission rates in 192 standard metropolitan statistical areas (SMSAs) controlling for the presence or absence of one or more HMOs in the state. His results indicated that the presence of an HMO in a state did correlate with a reduction in the overall admission rate in the state's SMSAs by an average 7.6 percent. However, it is not clear how the presence of an HMO in a state could affect rates in SMSAs that did not have an HMO.

Goldberg and Greenberg (1980) used multiple regression analysis to investigate the relationship between HMO market share and three measures of traditional insurers' response to HMOs: (1) federal employee nonmaternity days per 1,000 Blue Cross enrollees, (2) length of stay for maternity care for federal Blue Cross enrollees, and (3) hospital days per 1,000 Blue Cross nonfederal enrollees. They found that as the HMO market share increased in a state, all three measures declined. Hence, they concluded that higher HMO penetration in a state induced a competitive response from the Blue Cross plans who tightened their own utilization controls. However, this study was dominated by the experience of three west coast states and Hawaii. Therefore, the results may not hold across the nation.

It seems rather implausible that the state is the relevant market when trying to determine whether HMOs inject competition into a market. Since HMOs may be concentrated in only one or two SMSAs in a state, dividing a state's HMO enrollment by a state's population may not reflect the true impact of HMOs in the areas where they are most concentrated. Thus, more researchers have concentrated on (1) the SMSA, which represents an integrated social and economic system for the production and consumption of all market services, or (2) the areas served by Health Systems Agencies (HSA) which were established to be appropriate areas for the effective planning and development of health services.

McLaughlin et al. (1984) examined the impact of HMO penetration in twenty-five SMSAs on hospital admissions and hospital costs. They found that the average 6 percent market share of HMOs in the twenty-five SMSAs resulted in a 3 percent reduction in admission rates. However, they also found that as HMO enrollment increased in the SMSAs, hospital expenses per admission per day and per capita increased.

Minneapolis/St. Paul is believed to be a good area to test the competitive or "spill-over" effects of HMOs on the community because HMO enrollment there has increased dramatically over the last decade. Johnson and Aquilina (1986) found that HMOs in the Twin Cities had not significantly affected overall hospital costs, revenues or profits. In addition, they found no empirical evidence that HMOs had actively shopped for hospitals on the basis of price. Since HMOs obtained varying discounts from most hospitals, they developed some price insensitivity with regard to hospitals. Moreover, Johnson and Aquilina found that hospitals recouped their discounts to HMOs by raising their prices to non-HMO customers. As a result, the community did not experience any restraint in hospital finances.

In another study of the Twin Cities, Feldman et al. (1986) found that hospitals which gave discounts to HMOs and which had a large share of HMO patients did not have lower costs per admission than other hospitals. This finding suggests that discounts did not force hospitals to operate more efficiently. They also found that the costs of discounts to HMOs were shifted to other payers. Other research by McLaughlin (1987) and Merrill and McLaughlin (1986) tend to confirm these conclusions.

All of these studies point to the difficulty in isolating and measuring the effect of HMOs on health care costs. Many other factors in the health care market have been changing simultaneously with the growth of HMOs. The federal government has made greater efforts to control medicare and medicaid costs with DRGs. Other purchasers of health care are negotiating with hospitals and developing their own methods to control costs (e.g., preadmission certification, second opinions, and so on.). Also, nonhospital alternatives such as freestanding surgery centers have become substitutes for inpatient care.

Despite these problems in determining the competitive impact of HMOs, most research indicates that HMOs tend to have a negative impact on hospital admissions in a community. But their impact on hospital costs are not as clear. Perhaps it is not too surprising that HMOs would not have as great an impact on hospital costs. As HMOs reduce hospital admissions, the cases which are admitted to the hospital may be more serious and thus more expensive. Hence, even as admissions decline, hospital expenses per admission and per day may increase because of the more serious caseload.

HMOs are more likely to have an impact on a community if there is excess hospital capacity in the area. If there is minimal excess capacity, the hospitals have little reason to seek HMOs' business and to negotiate reduced rates. Likewise, if there is a shortage of physicians in an area, there will be little reason for physicians to participate in IPAs, accept more oversight, or adopt cost-conscious practices in treating fee-for-service patients. Since these physicians probably do not desire additional patients and can readily replace any lost to HMOs, they have little reason to accept the lower fees and strict controls that accompany IPA membership (Christianson 1980).

Unfortunately, HMOs do not always reward cost-containing behavior by directing patients to the cost-effective hospitals. Instead, they shop for discounts which are often passed on in the form of higher prices to other non-HMO purchasers. This further explains why greater HMO enrollment does not reduce hospital costs. Until HMOs comparison shop for comparable products and send their patients to cost-effective hospitals, a competition strategy to contain the rise in hospital costs probably will not be successful.

## PATIENT SELF-SELECTION BIAS

Patient self-selection is said to be biased when the premium payments for health care do not equal the actual costs because some factor about the insured population which affects utilization has not been considered in the calculation of the premium (Wilensky and Rossiter 1986). Bias is favorable when more healthy enrollees than expected enroll, and is adverse when higher than expected risks enroll.

Biased selection can lead to serious problems in the insurance market. If some plans consistently experience favorable selection, other plans may experience adverse selection and a poor financial condition as they serve an increasingly higher risk population. Increasing adverse selection ''could lead to a 'premium spiral' in which ever higher premiums must be paid by the least healthy segment of the population, defeating the purpose of insurance, which is to pool risk'' (Wilensky and Rossiter 1986, p. 67). The financial implications of biased selection make patient self-selection an important issue in the insurance industry, particularly for HMOs.

### Patient Choice Among Plans

Since self-selection by patients among plans determines whether biased selection occurs, it is well to know more about the factors involved in the choice. Perhaps the most important factor is perceived need for health care. There is a tendency to remain in whatever plan one is in if one does not anticipate much need for future care and if one's experiences in the plan have been satisfactory. Young single people often see little need for care and are indifferent to most factors except cost.

Those who have specific health needs will engage in a much more specific examination of plans and attempt to match their needs to anticipated benefits. They also desire freedom of choice and quality. These individuals are most averse to uncertainty and resist leaving physicians with whom they have a long established relationship. Indeed, an established doctor/patient relationship is very difficult to break even when there are significant cost advantages for the patient.

Another important factor is cost. Most consumers are cost sensitive and are attracted to plans that offer the lowest premiums and out-of-pocket expenses. Since the importance of cost varies in direct relationship to household income, low and modest income families will be more affected by costs.

Individuals will seek to shift health care plans when they feel dissatisfied with their present health care arrangements. Often the most crucial components of satisfaction are *access* and *physicians interest and responsiveness* (Mechanic 1990). The ability to make a timely appointment is a strong proxy for access. Waiting time in the office is also an important variable and affects groups differently. A highly paid professional typically has more sick leave, flexibility in hours and discretion than a manual worker paid near the minimum wage. Physical proximity to care and travel time are also components of access.

Patients are very interested in the physician's personal interest in them which explains why patients like to see the same doctor. Consumers seek good communication and the feeling that the doctor really cares about them. They don't like to feel rushed. Other variables that could affect choice decisions are attractiveness of facilities, amount of paperwork and forms, perceived responsiveness of support staff, availability of prevention and other special programs, and the use of a comprehensive hospital.

When considering these variables in making a choice among plans, consumers have little information. Indeed, most consumers have much more information about purchasing a car than they do about purchasing their health care. Thus, individuals can make choices that do not seem very rational given their own needs and preferences. Often, patients only obtain information by experience. This may explain why a larger percentage than average of a plan's population switch out of a plan very soon after enrollment. They find out that it was not what they had expected. Also, it may explain why patients are so hesitant to leave a doctor when they are relatively satisfied. They are reluctant to leave when the choices are difficult and uncertain. Moreover, the choices are probably even more difficult for those with less education and/or time to seek more information.

### Biased Selection and Employers Attitudes' about HMOs

As we saw earlier, HMOs tend to reduce utilization significantly. Yet employers have not uniformly embraced HMOs. A 1988 survey of large employers across the nation revealed that only 26 percent felt that their HMO premiums were fair (Foster Higgins 1988). This was down from 48 percent in 1987. The majority of respondents (54 percent) also felt that HMOs tended to attract the better risks (favorable selection) from their employee population and only a third felt that HMOs were effective in controlling health care costs.

Most larger employers either self-insure or have conventional experience-rated insurance plans. As a result, the premiums of these plans tend to reflect the costs incurred by those enrolled in the plans. In contrast, HMOs generally have used community ratings whereby premiums are based on costs incurred within the general community. Thus, if an HMO experiences favorable selection within a given employee group, its premiums for that group would not change very much since the premium is established by the community rate not the actual experience of the group. On the other hand, the adverse selection experienced by the conventional plan which contains the remaining higher-risk employees results in higher premiums (Luft and Miller 1988).

The problem was exacerbated when the employers based their contributions to the HMO on the cost of the fee-for-service option. Until recently, federal regulations required that employer payments to federally-qualified HMOs equal on a dollar to dollar basis those paid to the fee-for-service plan. If HMOs attracted low-risk people, and those who were high risk remained in the conventional plan, the employer had to contribute more to the conventional plans which in turn generated higher HMO premiums as well.

Employers have another reason to be concerned about higher-risk employees not selecting the HMO option. HMOs are intended to provide a cost-effective alternative in the delivery of health care. If the higher-risk employees who are most likely to have the more expensive sickness episodes are not in the most cost-efficient delivery system (an HMO) but instead remain in the more inefficient fee-for-service system, then the original intent behind HMOs is subverted.

## HMO Marketing/Enrollment Strategies and Biased Selection

Some believe HMOs use specific marketing strategies to attract lower risk enrollees, a process known as "risk skimming." For example, extensive well baby coverage attracts younger families but is not important to older couples who may have the more serious health problems. Thus, it encourages younger lower-risk people to join the HMO. A service like preventive dentistry is generally more attractive to a healthy population. Likewise, a sports medicine clinic is expressly designed to attract younger, more athletic enrollees who are among the lowest risks. On the other hand, offering complete drug coverage would attract a different group of enrollees. Since seniors with teeth intact are often healthier than their cohorts without teeth, a medicare dental supplemental plan could be designed to attract more healthy seniors (Luft and Miller 1988).

Premiums may be structured by HMOs so that family coverage is proportionately less expensive than individual coverage. As a result, families with children who tend to cost less per capita are attracted. Similarly, an HMO which has a large and excellent panel of primary care physicians, but a small, hard to reach group of specialists will tend to attract those who need primary care, but not acute, specialized, much more expensive care.

An HMO's facilities may likewise discourage those with higher risks. For example, if HMOs have a number of convenient, attractive outpatient care facilities, but few, if any, very large specialized hospitals, they may discourage enrollment of those who expect to use the more expensive treatments common in the large hospital. At the same time, they may attract the younger family with children who need the lower-cost outpatient services. Likewise, an HMO could be very purposeful about where it locates its clinics. Locating only in middle and upper income areas will tend to attract the more economically secure and healthier sections of the population.

HMOs may market their services by sponsoring get-acquainted socials at community events or through invitations to visit HMO facilities. Of course, such activities are much more likely to reach the more vigorous, active individuals rather than the homebound. Conversely, direct marketing by mail or telephone generally is not used by HMOs (Luft and Miller 1988).

HMOs may emphasize wellness programs and preventive medicine programs. While these are worthy and are to some extent implicit in the very concept of an HMO, they also appeal to a portion of the population that tends to practice more healthy living habits. Similarly, such individuals often are more conservative in their use of medicine. They may believe that the "natural," self-healing approach is best. Whether such an approach is better or not, it is certainly less expensive.

By all of these techniques and others, HMOs can encourage biased enrollment that produces favorable selection into HMOs. Moreover, the biased selection need not be very large to have a considerable economic impact. Studies reveal that one percent of the population accounts for 25 percent of the costs (Newhouse 1986). Thus, if HMOs are moderately successful in discouraging enrollment by the high cost few, they could reap considerable economic rewards.

## Evidence of Biased Selection in HMOs

A number of studies have examined whether biased selection exists in HMOs. Most studies look at the choice between one HMO option and a fee-for-service option. There are considerable methodological problems with a number of these studies. It is unclear how the inclusion of people facing multiple choices instead of just two could affect predictions of selection bias. Moreover, there are certain factors such as propensity to consume health services that cannot be directly observed and which affect health plan choice and use. In addition, there is anticipated need for services. For example, a family with generally low use of health care could anticipate higher health care needs and move from a plan with a low premium but high copayment to a more comprehensive HMO. In addition, most studies do not include all relevant variables in the health plan choice such as the distance to an HMO or waiting time to see a physician (Hellinger 1987).

Researchers sometimes studied a nonrandom sample of plans and studied some markets, but not others. HMO characteristics varied widely from newness of the plan to how long it had been offered to a group. They differed in market penetration and in the degree of competition from other HMOs and traditional insurance plans. Likewise, HMO premiums and benefits relative to traditional fee-for-service plans varied widely.

Despite those problems in the studies, the literature does indicate significant patterns of selection bias. Table 3.2 provides a summary of twenty-one self-selection studies between 1974 and 1986 that are reviewed by Wilensky and Rossiter (1986). Only three studies found adverse selection into an HMO, while eight found either no evidence of biased selection or were inconclusive. However, ten of the studies found evidence of favorable selection into the HMOs.

Luft and Miller (1988) also reviewed a number of selection studies which compared enrollees in HMOs with those in traditional plans on the basis of (1) prior health care use, (2) prior health care costs, and (3) health status. The results of Luft and Miller's review are summarized in Tables 3.3 and 3.4.

When comparing new HMO enrollees with non-HMO enrollees (Table 3.3), it is clear that HMOs attract individuals with the same or lower health care use and costs than non-HMO enrollees. While there is an apparent trend of favorable selection into HMOs, the evidence is not overwhelming. Fourteen of the twenty-two observations on prior use and eight of eighteen observations on prior cost show no difference or show adverse selection into HMOs. In addition, the favorable selection results may be exaggerated if new HMO enrollees have "stored-up" health care use just prior to joining the HMO in anticipation of the HMO's more comprehensive benefits (Luft and Miller 1988).

Health status in these studies is generally a self-report measure in which enrollees are asked to assess their health across a number of dimensions. While the validity of these self-reports may be open to some criticism, they do not indicate the level of favorable selection into HMOs found in prior health care use and costs. In fact, of the 13 observations of health status and enrollment in Luft and Miller's review, four show adverse selection into HMOs, eight show neutral results and only one favorable selection (See Table 3.3). Thus, HMOs may enroll people of roughly similar health status as those in traditional plans, but HMOs may enroll few or fewer of the small group of very sick people who constitute much of the use and costs of any plan (Luft and Miller 1988).

These studies tend to show that those who have used less health care tend to join HMOs. These individuals often are younger, lower-risk people who may be new to a community and who have fewer ties to medical care providers. On the other hand, those who do not join are those who have used more health care and thus have ties with physicians and hospitals. They are more concerned about the possible need to sever these ties if they joined an HMO. Attachments to physicians is perhaps the most important reason why people do not join HMOs. Juba, Lave, and Shaddy (1980) state that "integration in the local medical care system is a dominant factor in the decision to select a particular health plan. . . . Families having strong well-established ties with personal physicians will opt for an insurance plan that preserves these associations." With this fact in mind, it is not surprising that those with well-developed ties to physicians would be particularly reluctant to join a PGP type HMO with its limited panel of doctors.

**Table 3.2**
**Patient Self-Selection Studies**

| Study | Year | Population | Measurement | Findings |
|---|---|---|---|---|
| Bice | 1975 | Low-income families | Preenrollment claims | HMO adverse selection |
| Hetherington, Hopkins, Roemer | 1975 | Employment-based | Chronic health problems | HMO adverse selection |
| Tessler, Mechanic | 1975 | Employment-based | Chronic health problems | HMO adverse selection |
| Berki, Ashcraft Penchansky, Fortus | 1977 | Employment-based | Self-reported health status | No evidence for biased selection |
| Scitovsky, McCall, Benham | 1978 | Employment-based | Self-reported health status | No evidence for biased selection |
| Eggers | 1980 | Medicare | Preenrollment service use | HMO favorable selection |
| Juba, Lave, Shaddy | 1980 | Employment-based | Chronic health problems | Not conclusive |
| McGuire | 1981 | Employment-based | Years of age | Not conclusive |
| Eggers, Prihoda | 1982 | Medicare | Prior service use | HMO favorable selection |
| Jackson-Beeck, Klein | 1983 | Employment-based | Preenrollment claims | HMO favorable selection |
| Price, Mays, Trapnell | 1983 | Employment-based | Premium changes | HMO favorable selection |
| Welch, Frank, Diehr | 1984 | Employment-based | Service use and imputed costs | Not conclusive |
| Dowd, Feldman | 1985 | Employment-based | Chronic health problems | HMO favorable selection |
| Ellis | 1985 | Employment-based | Prior year enrollment claims | Not conclusive |
| Farley, Monheit | 1985 | Employment-based | Expenditures and premiums | No evidence for biased selection |
| Lubitz, Beebe, Riley | 1985 | Medicare | Medicare claims, service use | Not conclusive |
| Luft, Trauner, Maerki | 1985 | Retired employee | Age-sex distribution | HMO favorable selection |
| Price, May | 1985 | Employment-based | Premium changes over time | HMO favorable selection |
| Welch | 1985 | Medicare | Preenrollment claims | HMO favorable selection but declines |
| Merrill, Jackson, Reuter | 1985 | Employment-based | Prior year enrollment claims | HMO favorable selection |
| Buchanan, Cretin | 1986 | Employment-based | Prior claims | HMO favorable selection |

*Source*: G. Wilensky and L. Rossiter. "Patient Self-Selection in HMOs." *Health Affairs* 5 (1986): 70. Reprinted with permission.

* Almost All favorable Section Studies use prior use - But, if people are joining mostly for cost savings then there is a greater chance they used less srvcs before because they couldn't afford them.

**Table 3.3**
**Selection Bias Results for Different HMO Types, New HMO Enrollees Versus Non-HMO Enrollees**

| | Number of selection bias observations | | | | | | | | |
|---|---|---|---|---|---|---|---|---|---|
| | Prior Use | | | Prior Cost | | | Health status | | |
| HMO Type | Fav. | Neu. | Unfav. | Fav. | Neu. | Unfav. | Fav. | Neu. | Unfav. |
| Prepaid group practice | 5 | 3 | 0 | 6 | 2 | 0 | 1 | 2 | 3 |
| IPA | 2 | 4 | 1 | 2 | 3 | 1 | 0 | 4 | 0 |
| Don't know/both | 1 | 4 | 2 | 2 | 2 | 0 | 0 | 2 | 1 |

*Source*: H. S. Luft and R. H. Miller. "Patient Self-Selection in A Competitive Health Care System." *Health Affairs* 7 (1988): 107. Reprinted with permission.

*Note*: Fav. = favorable; Neu. = neutral; Unfav. = unfavorable to the HMO.

**Table 3.4**
**Selection Bias Results For Different HMO Types, Disenrollment Observations**

| | Number of selection bias observations | | | | | | | | |
|---|---|---|---|---|---|---|---|---|---|
| | Use | | | Cost | | | Health status | | |
| HMO Type | Fav. | Neu. | Unfav. | Fav. | Neu. | Unfav. | Fav. | Neu. | Unfav. |
| Prepaid group practice | 1 | 1 | 6 | 0 | 0 | 0 | 0 | 0 | 2 |
| IPA | 1 | 0 | 0 | 0 | 0 | 0 | 0 | 0 | 0 |
| Don't know/both | 0 | 0 | 1 | 3 | 1 | 0 | 0 | 0 | 0 |
| Total | 2 | 1 | 7 | 3 | 1 | 0 | 0 | 0 | 2 |

*Source*: H. S. Luft and R. H. Miller. "Patient Self-Selection in a Competitive Health Care System." *Health Affairs* 7 (1988): 109. Reprinted with permission.

*Note*: Fav. = Favorable; Neu. = neutral; Unfav. = unfavorable to the HMO.

However, such individuals might be more willing to join an IPA which includes a wider selection of physicians. Indeed, the IPA might include their old fee-for-service physician. PGPs are more likely than IPAs to attract those who have lower health utilization, lower health costs, and fewer ties to the medical system. As a result, PGPs tend to experience more favorable selection than IPAs (See Table 3.2). This fact should be remembered when comparing the ability of PGPs and IPAs to control health care costs.

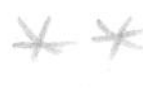

## Disenrollment in HMOs

Biased selection in HMOs could not only result from nonrandom selection of new enrollees, but also from nonrandom disenrollment. In other words, are those who leave HMOs more likely to be high users or low users of medical care? This is an important question since annual disenrollment rates in HMOs can reach 20 percent or higher.

One should note that there are several reasons for disenrollment. Mandatory disenrollment occurs when an individual moves out of the HMO service area or changes employers and the new employer does not offer the HMO. Disenrollment could occur because of a change in the relative prices, benefits and quality of the HMO and the FFS option.

Disenrollment could also occur because some believe they made a mistake in joining an HMO. Research reveals that those who receive the most information about an HMO before they join it are the most likely to be satisfied with the HMO and unlikely to leave it (Andrews et al. 1989). Those who joined an HMO without much information may be particularly likely to be disappointed. This is even more true for new HMOs. In long established HMOs, one can assess how well one will like it by talking to current members.

Luft and Miller (1988) found in their review of studies on HMO disenrollment that the prior use of health care for HMO disenrollees was less than that of those HMO enrollees who elected to stay in the HMO. This was true in seven of eight studies (See Table 3.4). Some of these studies failed to control for out-of-plan use by the disenrollees. Mechanic et al. (1983) and Wollstadt et al. (1978) found out-of-plan visits of leavers to be much higher than that of stayers. Low use of HMO services combined with higher out-of-plan visits and subsequent disenrollment could indicate dissatisfaction with the HMO. Also, such out-of-plan use may explain why Luft and Miller found that after disenrollment HMO disenrollees had higher health care use or health care costs than did fee-for-service enrollees.

These studies tend to indicate that those who leave HMOs tend to be those who use less health services. Welch (1985) has estimated that leavers have 15 percent fewer visits (based on studies using out-of-plan utilization) and 40 percent fewer hospital days. Thus, while HMOs experience favorable selection of new enrollees, they tend to suffer adverse disenrollment. Why? First, those who leave may never have been integrated into the HMO system. They did not have ties to HMO physicians and thus saw little to lose in leaving. Second, some may have voluntarily deferred utilization until leaving the HMO in order to obtain physicians and hospitals unavailable in the HMOs. If so, this would explain why those who disenroll from an HMO seem to use less health care than those who remain in the HMO but more than those who are in the fee-for-service plan. They "stored-up" health care use until they left the HMO. Some disenrollment may result from HMO enrollees who need surgical or specialty care but who want these performed by physicians outside the HMO whom they had known before joining the HMO. Therefore, it is possible that some adverse disenrollment from HMOs is, paradoxically, also adverse enrollment for traditional fee-for-service plans.

These studies still leave some questions unanswered. Few studies have investigated the selection effects of new plans (less than three years old) with those for older, more established plans (Wrightson 1990). New plans tend to attract lower-risk employees who do not have established physician ties that must be broken to join the new plan. Likewise, few studies have been done on the selection effects experienced by both established HMOs and an indemnity plan when a new HMO is introduced.

Few studies have studied the cumulative effects of a favorable or unfavorable "selection spiral" (Wrightson 1990). If an indemnity plan suffers unfavorable selection, the plan is left with more and more higher-risk individuals which force the premiums even higher. Conversely, if a plan experienced favorable selection would its rates also tend to spiral (i.e., would the rates tend to decrease or remain less than inflation as more and more low-risk individuals were attracted to the plan)?

### Impact of Favorable Selection into HMOs

The impact of favorable selection into HMOs may not be as great as would first appear. There is evidence in several studies that new HMO enrollees have "stored" health care needs before they enroll. Thus, they appear to be low utilizers. However, there is also evidence that those who disenroll from HMOs may also "store" health care needs. Thus, the "leavers" behavior in the year prior to leaving one plan and enrolling in another may not be particularly representative of the individual's actual use of health care across several years.

There is evidence for this assumption in several studies. Lubitz et al. (1985) found that health expenses are not related over time, even among the high-risk elderly. While a plan may attract low-risk enrollees at first, in several years costs for the enrolled population will increase (Welch 1985). Thus, "regression toward the mean" suggests that in time both lower and higher than average risks move toward the mean risk experience (Riley et al. 1989).

While HMOs enjoy favorable enrollment, they also suffer adverse disenrollment. Hence, over time there may be a balancing effect. Preferential enrollment and adverse disenrollment together suggest that the well tend to move between plans and the sick tend to stay where they are (Welch 1985). The effects of favorable and unfavorable selection tend to deteriorate over time and plans respond to this change and the market through premium adjustments.

New HMOs, recently presented to a group of employees, are most likely to experience favorable selection. Given the halt in the development of new HMOs since 1987, this situation is much less likely to occur. Also, the increased flexibility in HMO rate setting permitted by the 1988 amendments to the HMO Act removes many of the incentives for HMOs trying to enroll low-risk employees (See Chapter 5). Since federally qualified HMOs are now permitted to use a form of experience rating, employers can pressure HMOs to base their rates on the specific historical health care experience of their employees. Therefore, the HMO would lose much of its incentive to seek out the low risks.

The main problem of biased selection in a competitive market with more and more options for enrollees is that plans place too much emphasis on techniques of marketing to attract low risk groups instead of improving efficiency. Likewise, in such an environment, much more emphasis may be placed on attempts to encourage high-risk individuals to leave the plan. As a result, marketing and promotional efforts might become excessive, costly, dysfunctional, and could jeopardize quality and efficiency (Wilensky and Rossiter 1986). Employers have a major responsibility to mitigate these tendencies, which is the subject of the next section.

## CONTROLLING BIASED SELECTION

If employers hope to deal effectively with HMOs or any insurance plan, they must have data. They must follow their employees' enrollment patterns. However, the difficulty in developing enrollee specific measures is underscored by the fact that many employers do not know exactly how many dependents their employees have. Nevertheless, employers must know more about predictors of health care use in order to evaluate premiums.

Employers should first compare the demographic data of employees enrolled in the different plans. There are rough correlations among gender, age, marital status and family size and health care costs. Thus, employers should know whether their HMOs tend to attract those employees who are demographically lower risks.

Prior medical care utilization data (e.g., hospitalization, physician visits, tests, prescriptions) is often the best predictor of future use. Therefore, employers should compare such data with similar data for employees in the non-HMO plan and with other groups in the HMO. Remember that utilization data, not costs, should receive the initial focus. Otherwise, an HMO may be accused of skimming because of its lower costs when the real reason for the lower costs was greater efficiency.

Certain measures of health status derived from questionnaires have predicted health care use across different types of delivery systems (Thomas et al. 1983, Manning et al. 1982). Employers could use some of these devices to explore which employees are likely to be higher risks. All of this information is sought to better allow the employer to accurately predict health care utilization and costs for a particular group of employees.

Employers should also be sure that "apples-to-apples" comparisons are used when comparing plan utilization data and costs. Employers should be particularly attentive to what and who is covered in the plans. Some employers have learned that HMOs have not allowed enrollment of some employees who are covered by the indemnity plan. For example, some HMOs have not covered permanently disabled former employees who are covered by the indemnity plan. Similar exclusions could occur for early retirees, widows, divorced spouses and part-time employees (Halvorson 1988). Failure to provide coverage to such groups could seriously distort utilization and cost comparisons.

Recent changes in federal legislation allows HMOs to use more flexible rating systems (See Chapter 5). As a result, employers, particularly large ones, with substantial negotiating leverage can pressure HMOs to use adjusted community rating (ACR) or community rating by class (CRC) rather than community rating (CR) when establishing rates for employees (Anderson et al. 1986). ACR or CRC can better estimate the expected costs of providing care to a specific group of employees than can CR, and thus can partially offset the costs of skimming by an HMO.

Employers should be careful that they are not victims of "predatory pricing" and "shadow pricing" (Halvorson 1988). These occur when an HMO offers an initial low-cost premium which is designed to appeal to lower-risk employees. Once the lower-risk employees join the HMO, the higher-risk employees become more concentrated in the non-HMO plan. As a result, it has to increase its premium dramatically. After a year or so, the HMO, pointing to the price increases of its competition, announces that it too must raise its rates significantly to a point just below the competition (i.e., shadow pricing). An employer must use good utilization data to confront and defeat this tactic.

Employers can also use utilization data and cost data to negotiate different rates in different cities. It may be unwise for a large national employer to pay a single national premium or capitation rate to an HMO. Health care costs can differ dramatically in different cities and regions. Paying an "average" national rate to an HMO could result in premiums that were considerably higher than the average indemnity plan costs in the less expensive cities. Conversely, in the more expensive cities, the national average would be low resulting in greater portions of the HMO premium being covered by the employees. In such a situation, most employees would probably remain with the old indemnity plan. As a result, the employer pays more for health care in the less expensive cities which is not balanced by compensating savings in the more expensive ones.

Similarly, if an employer has different units which employ very different types of employees, it might be best to break out insurance costs for each unit (Halvorson 1988). For example, if one unit has nearly all white collar employees with comparatively low health care use, while another unit has heavy manufacturing employees with higher medical care costs, it may be preferable to have separate HMO contracts for each group rather than have one average rate for both units. By having different contracts for each unit, the employer can negotiate rates that are more likely to encourage the higher-risk employees in the manufacturing unit to join an HMO.

Employers should give more consideration to the enrollment strategies of indemnity plans, HMOs and other options (Halvorson 1988). Since the employers purchase health care plans, they can have much influence over how the plans are presented to their employees. Employers can insist that their personnel staffs explain the benefits and costs of all options. Thus, employers can take special steps to see that HMOs do not engage in skimming and that the benefits of HMOs are presented to higher-risk employees. In this vein, employers should probably do much more to describe the benefits and costs of competing plans to employees. Brochures, films, and other media that discuss the quality, access and cost of the various health insurance plans should be provided.

If an employer concludes that an HMO has experienced favorable selection and is skimming its employees, and if the HMO refuses to negotiate rates based on actual experience, then the employer might consider other strategies to balance the risks (Dowd and Feldman 1985). The employer could offer a very austere and inexpensive indemnity plan to lure low-risk employees back from the HMO and also to reduce the attractiveness of the indemnity plan to the higher utilizers. Thus, an employer could offer an austere indemnity plan that features higher coinsurance, higher deductibles and more out-of-pocket expenses for most services, but provide complete coverage for preventive care, maternity care and other services attractive to low-risk employees. The goal in this strategy is not to favor one plan over another but to balance risk groups appropriately (Halvorson 1988).

Another approach that an employer could use to reduce skimming is to eliminate the separate risk pools by offering an HMO with an open, point of service, or choice plan. Under such a plan, the enrollees make a choice, at the point of service, to stay fully covered within the network of HMO providers or to seek care outside of the network and pay a deductible and coinsurance. Benefits are generally less outside of the network and deductibles are $200 to $400 with coinsurance of 20 to 30 percent.

The obvious advantage of such plans to employers is that the HMO takes all the risk and has incentives to move high-risk individuals into the more economical HMO network. Indeed, more and more employers are concluding that the best way to control biased selection is to use an open point of service choice plan as a "total replacement" for all health plans (Halvorson 1988). HMOs offer such plans to remain competitive, to address employers' concerns about skimming, and because most believe that they can keep use of non-HMO providers to under 10 to 15 percent.

Wrightson (1990) has identified several factors that can affect the success of the "total replacement" or "sole sourcing" arrangement. First, the HMO must offer experience-based premiums. Thus, the employer and the HMO have every incentive to encourage all employees to use the HMO services. Second, the HMO should be well-known and respected by employees and have a proven track record in the community. The higher the percentage of employees covered by the HMO at the time of sole sourcing, the higher the likelihood of success. Third, the HMO must have ample physicians and facilities which are conveniently located for most employees. Fourth, the employer must be willing to market and sell the HMO to its employees. Even though there is freedom of choice with the arrangement, there will be some initial employee dissatisfaction which the employer must anticipate. Finally, transition assistance in the form of orientation meetings, written material and telephone hot lines which explain the new program must be provided. If these conditions are present, ''sole sourcing'' may be the best prescription for both real and suspicioned biased selection.

As employers become more sophisticated and use a variety of the approaches noted above to control biased selection, whatever skimming occurs by HMOs (which is probably considerably less than most employers suspicion), will become less and less significant.

Of course, it is entirely possible that an HMO could experience adverse selection and enroll a disproportionate number of higher-risk, more costly employees. In such a situation, the employer should take considerable care to see that the HMO continues to enroll these employees and that the HMO continues its contract. HMOs can be a real asset in cost containment, particularly if they enroll the less healthy employees. Therefore, employers should consider increasing their contributions to any HMO that is suffering adverse selection. If such an HMO decided to stop doing business with the employer, the higher-risk employees would probably return to the indemnity plan which would almost certainly be much more costly to the employer.

## CONCLUSION

HMOs' ability to control costs is not as great as originally hoped nor as impotent as critics suggest. The evidence is clear that HMOs, particularly PGPs, can reduce hospitalization. In turn, this decrease reduces premiums and out-of-pocket costs for HMO enrollees. However, these savings occur only once. Afterward, HMOs experience cost increases slightly lower than or very similar to those of traditional insurers.

HMOs have not been able to translate reduction in hospitalization into overall or community wide reduction in hospital costs. As noted earlier, HMOs often are more interested in obtaining discounts than in shopping for hospitals that offer the least expensive prices. More importantly, hospitals compensate for discounts by raising the price for other buyers. Thus, overall hospital costs or costs per patient, or costs per capita may go up even as hospitalization decreases. Hence, the competitive effects of HMOs on health care costs for non-HMO enrollees appear to be few and weak.

The success of HMOs has been questioned by those who claim HMOs experience favorable enrollment. Although HMOs do often attract those who are healthier, the effect is probably not as great as many critics and employers believe. While HMOs attract low risk enrollees, they also lose low-risks through disenrollment. Thus, favorable selection and adverse disenrollment may cancel each other out. The more pernicious effects of biased selection may occur as HMOs try to concentrate too much on marketing and attracting low-risks instead of achieving real efficiencies.

Before HMOs will be effective in reducing costs, employers must become more knowledgeable and forceful in their negotiations with HMOs. Employers must push for more experience ratings from HMOs in order to capture more of the savings from HMOs' lower utilization. Even after such changes, however, HMOs can provide only limited respite from continuing cost increases as long as Americans' desire for more and more health care, whatever its utility, outpaces their distaste of its costs.

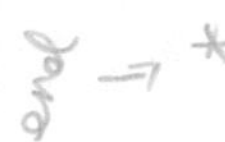

# 4

# Quality in HMOs

As the drive for cost-containment in HMOs accelerates, there is increased concern about the quality of care provided by HMOs. Thus, patients and employers are increasingly asking HMOs to document their efforts to promote quality care. As a result, more and more HMOs understand that their quality assurance processes are useful in both improving their organizations and in marketing their health care products.

## DEFINITION OF QUALITY

A recent survey of physicians, consumers, and employers reveals the many and various definitions of quality (Kechley Report 1988). Employers tended to define quality in terms of medical care outcomes. They believed that outcomes were related to how often a hospital or physician performed a particular procedure, the training of the medical staff, and the availability of care. Consumers believed that quality indicated good doctors and modern equipment and facilities. They thought good doctors were those who stayed up-to-date, kept patients informed, and treated patients with dignity. The physicians believed that quality was a result of physicians' training, the availability of competent nurses, the technical capacity of the facilities, and the quality of physician/patient relations.

These various views of quality reflect the three major measures of quality—structural, process, and outcome measures. Structural measures refer to those "inputs" into the medical care system that are believed to favorably affect medical outcomes. Such structural factors include characteristics of providers such as training, certification, and membership in medical societies. Also included are staffing ratios, availability of technical equipment, and accreditation of hospitals.

Process measures of quality refer to the review of medical records by medical experts to determine if the proper treatment was provided in a particular episode of illness.

Outcome measures attempt to assess what actually happens to the patient or the end results of medical care. Outcome measures might include levels of mortality, morbidity, blood pressure, and other indices of health status.

## Structural Measures of Quality

Structural measures do not actually measure the quality of health outcomes. They only measure an environment or the ingredients that experts believe to be conducive to quality. Luft's (1981) review of structural quality studies indicates that the quality of medical care in HMOs is at least as good, and perhaps better, than it is in the FFS sector. HMOs tend to have higher proportions of board-certified specialists and are more likely to use qualified surgeons (Luft 1981).

HMOs have a formal organizational structure that, other things being equal, tend to promote more peer review and more formal and informal consultation among physicians in the group. Since HMOs establish requirements that providers must meet in order to join the HMO, one can assume that quality may be higher as compared to independent solo practitioners in the FFS system. Likewise, an HMO is more likely to take faster action against poor performance than might occur among solo practitioners in the FFS system.

HMOs emphasize efforts in continuing education. Similarly, most HMOs have internal quality review procedures. Both of these structural factors should encourage quality.

Donabedian (1983) believes certain structural properties of HMOs could permit them to be quality leaders. They serve a defined population which leads to greater accountability for output. They provide more comprehensive care which encourages greater continuity of care. Finally, they provide care through a formally organized effort which provides for integration of efforts.

Likewise, Bates and Brown (1988) found that HMO technologies enhanced care. The more organized relationships among providers in HMOs, particularly in staff and group-model HMOs, enhanced the continuity and coordination needed for the chronic care needs of the elderly. In addition, the emphasis on ambulatory care in HMOs reduced the threat of intrusive practice patterns that contributed only marginally to the diagnosis and management of illness.

Finally, most HMOs have health promotion programs. A recent survey reveals that approximately 75 percent of HMOs provide at least one wellness activity (Bernton 1987). Wellness activities included are smoking cessation, weight loss, stress management, hypertension reduction, and programs to control drug and alcohol abuse. While HMOs offer these programs primarily as a marketing service, they nevertheless may have a positive impact on the quality of health. These structural assessments indicate that the quality of care in HMOs is at least as good and perhaps better than it is in the FFS sector.

It should be noted that these structural elements of HMOs which appear reasonably related to quality are most pronounced in staff or group-model HMOs. The fast growing open-panel IPAs which accept most doctors who apply and which contract directly with many individual doctors may lack many of these structural and organizational elements. Further, these IPAs may often lack the collegial and professional peer interaction which enhances quality in group or staff-model HMOs. Finally, if such IPAs place individual doctors rather than *groups* of doctors directly at risk for overutilization, quality may be compromised for the direct economic benefits of lower utilization. (For more discussion of this concern, see Chapter 6.)

## Process Measures of Quality

Process measures evaluate the process of care to determine if the most appropriate care was given. However, evaluating the process of care in most cases "requires explicit criteria that the medical profession (or other provider groups) agree are relevant, important and measurable" (Lohr et al. 1988, 11). Such measures should be reliable and valid or produce the same result when the same case is measured again, and they should measure what they purport to measure. Unfortunately, there is no comprehensive inventory of all the diagnosis-specific criteria that could be used today (Lohr et al. 1988). Thus, it is not easy to statistically confirm the reliability and validity of many process measures.

Luft's extensive review of process studies (1981) indicated that HMOs provided care equal to or superior to the average FFS practitioner. Subsequent process studies tend to confirm this conclusion. Yelin et al. (1986) conducted a two-year study of the care of rheumatoid arthritis patients in prepaid settings and in FFS arrangements. They found that the prepaid patients received similar amounts and kinds of health care as their fee-for-service counterparts. Francis et al. (1984) also found similar care in the treatment of colorectal cancer in patients in HMO and FFS settings. There were no differences in definitive surgery, chemotherapy, radiation therapy, length of hospitalization and number of follow-up physician visits.

Langwell and Hadley (1989) found that HMO and FFS physicians provided very similar treatment of congestive heart failure and colorectal cancer. However, in terms of more routine care, they found that HMO providers were more likely to take better medical histories, provide more complete physical examinations, more screening tests and a greater frequency of immunizations than did FFS providers (Langwell and Hadley 1989). Thus, it appears that HMOs do at least as well as FFS providers on process measures.

## Outcome Measures of Quality

Outcome measures attempt to measure the end result of health care—that is, the actual health status of the patient. While such measurement seems inherently the most logical approach to evaluation of quality, it is used much less than the other approaches. Luft notes (1981, 209) that "the difficulty arises from an inability to measure health status on a sufficiently fine and accurate scale to identify small but important differences." Moreover, measures such as mortality may represent only a small part of the true outcome of care.

Outcome measures require a great amount of data that is not easy to acquire. Moreover, it is difficult to make comparisons among outcome data because the case mix of the patients compared may be different. Some patients may consult a physician too late in the progress of a disease. Another problem is that outcome measures usually judge outcomes according to what providers think are important (i.e., mortality, morbidity, etc.) rather than what the patients want. Some patients may, for example, prefer a different lifestyle (such as a different diet or drugs) in exchange for some decline in mortality. As a result of these problems, many physicians resist the use of outcome measures. They most often prefer that the appropriateness of their actions rather than their effects be judged.

After a review of specific outcome data for particular diseases in both FFS and HMO settings, Luft (1981) concluded that the outcomes for HMOs were about the same as for FFS providers. Subsequent data tend to confirm this conclusion. Francis et al. (1984) found that colorectal cancer patients treated by HMOs and FFS providers had the same outcomes as measured by four year survival rates and one year health status. After two years of follow-up, Yelin et al. (1986) found similar outcomes for rheumatoid arthritis patients in HMO and FFS settings.

Some outcome measures evaluate broad health status outcomes rather than outcomes for specific diseases. These broad outcome measures include functional status and physical capacity measures, mental health inventories, and measures of a person's perceptions of his or her general health (Brook and Lohr 1985). Ware et al. (1986) studied the health status of patients in an HMO and in an FFS setting. Health status was measured by 13 indices. They found that after 3 to 5 years, the health outcomes for higher-income patients were significantly better in the HMO. However, the low-income patients tended to do better in the FFS system. On the other hand, Sloss et al. (1987) looked at the same groups as did Ware but used a different set of 25 health status measures. They found no significant differences between the low-income individuals in the FFS and HMO groups. Another study by Marcus and Stone (1984) found no differences in morbidity between FFS and HMO patients.

In a longitudinal study of health status outcomes of Medicare beneficiaries in FFS settings and in HMOs, Langwell and Hadley (1989) found no significant differences between the two groups in the percent of beneficiaries whose health status had worsened between baseline and follow-up surveys and no significant differences in the percent who showed no change in health status. Thus, these outcome studies, like the structural and process studies, reveal that HMOs do at least as well as FFS providers in providing quality medical care.

**Summary of Quality Measures**

Unfortunately, quality measures in health care continue to leave much to be desired. While structural and process measures remain the dominant methods of measurement, they are not direct indicators of the health status of patients. Moreover, they do not correlate well with most outcome measures. Thus, they may not be truly important in the improvement of long-term health.

On the other hand, outcome measures may not be valid or they may be unable to discern the true impact of structural and process variables. In addition, outcome studies may not adequately control for differences in patients when they entered the health care system. Indeed, this is a primary reason why many medical care providers are reluctant to use outcome measures. They believe that there are often significant differences in the case mix of comparison groups of patients. Hence, providers often suggest that the outcome measures may be measuring differences in patients, not effectiveness of treatment.

Despite these problems with structural, process, and outcome measures, they are the only ones available at this time. From these measures, it appears that HMOs can provide a quality of health care that is at least as good and perhaps better than that provided by the average FFS provider.

There is some evidence that HMOs may not move as rapidly as FFS providers in providing definitive care to patients (Francis et al. 1984). This probably results from HMOs' conservative approach and hesitancy to hospitalize. Similarly, HMOs may be less inclined to use as many tests as FFS providers. For example, Epstein et al. (1986) found that patients with uncomplicated hypertension received 50 percent more electrocardiograms from FFS providers than from HMOs, and 40 percent more chest radiographs. FFS doctors believed that both tests were associated with high profits.

Since HMOs have an economic incentive in taking a slower or more conservative approach, they may be particularly unlikely to overly prescribe treatment for the "worried well." They may reassure patients that their symptoms are self-limiting or part of the normal aging process (Hornbook and Berki 1985). Conversely, HMOs may be less quick to diagnose and treat the "subtly sick," who may not be distinguishable from the worried well by only a routine clinical examination (Hornbook and Berki 1985). The demands of the subtly sick may appear unreasonable to some HMO physicians. They may be reluctant to order more tests and thus may adopt a "wait and see" strategy rather than an aggressive diagnostic strategy. These subtly sick patients may have poor outcomes in the more conservative HMO practice environment where laboratory tests (Epstein et al. 1986) and referrals (Luke and Thomson 1980) may be less likely to occur. In the aggregate, the effect of a conservative strategy does not appear to affect health outcomes. However, it could be detrimental in the case of some diseases where early detection and treatment are critical to successful outcomes.

## CONSUMER SATISFACTION

Consumer satisfaction with the quality of care may be the ultimate test of quality. Certainly, patient satisfaction is critical to the success of HMOs in an increasingly competitive health care marketplace. Thus, HMOs and employers must be very concerned about how the consumers evaluate medical care delivery. Most satisfaction surveys include sections on satisfaction with access, availability, continuity of care, humanness, information transfer, quality and overall satisfaction.

### Concern About Consumer Surveys

Although patient or consumer satisfaction surveys appear to be a vital part of the evaluation of health care delivery, they continue to receive considerable criticism. Critics argue that data from consumers (1) reveal more about the consumer than the quality of care, (2) reflect the quantity of health care rather than the quality, (3) do not correlate with physicians' judgment of quality, and (4) simply reflect the friendliness of providers not their technical skills (Davies and Ware 1988).

Because consumers' ratings of the quality of medical care may correlate with their educational level, age, income, ethnicity, attitudes toward the community, satisfaction with life, and their expectation regarding medical care, some critics question their validity as assessments of medical care (Linn and Greenfield 1982; Linn et al. 1984). This argument assumes, however, that all associations between these consumer attributes and medical care reflect bias. This may not be true. For example, medical care may be delivered differently to people of different ages or races or income. Indeed, the evidence used to support this criticism comes from correlational studies in which the quality of medical care was unknown or not held constant (Davies and Ware 1988).

Experimental studies that have changed the elements of medical encounters for individuals who were randomly assigned to view the encounters have not found significant associations among the ratings of medical care and personal attributes (Davies and Ware 1988). "Thus results from several studies suggest that bias from personal characteristics is minimal for technical quality. Taken together, the available evidence does not support the conclusion that this bias is strong enough to invalidate consumers' ratings of the quality of their care" (Davies and Ware 1988, 36).

Some critics of consumer surveys suggest that consumers can be seduced by the number of tests and services performed by doctors into believing that they received high quality care. Studies do reveal that consumers' ratings of quality do tend to correlate with quantity (Sox et al. 1981). This tendency to confuse more with good may tend to bias consumer surveys against HMOs which make concerted efforts to control the quantity of care and to take a conservative approach to care.

Critics also suggest that consumer judgments of quality are not valid because they do not correlate with the expert judgments of doctors. Of course, this criticism overlooks the fact that physicians often do not share identical judgments of technical quality (Eddy 1984). Moreover, studies do indicate that consumers' evaluations of technical quality do agree with physicians for common problems (Davies and Ware 1988). Also, physicians and consumers tend to agree more about what constitutes *poor* care, which is the critical concern of most quality assurance efforts.

Finally, critics suggest that consumers' attitudes about the interpersonal aspects of care affect their judgments of its quality. Of course, the correlational studies which show this association did not control the technical delivery of care. Thus, the quality of technical care may indeed have varied along with changes in the interpersonal relationship. Other studies which have experimentally controlled the technical quality of care while changing the interpersonal aspects have found that interpersonal aspects had an insignificant effect on technical quality ratings (Davies and Ware 1988). Thus, it appears that at least for more common medical care, patients can separate their ratings of the technical quality of care from their ratings of the interpersonal aspects of care.

### Reasons for Using Consumer Surveys

Several reasons for conducting consumer surveys are: (1) consumers' assessments of quality are valid indicators of their choice of health plans and options in the healthcare market; (2) consumers can provide valid data about quality; (3) consumer survey data are less expensive to collect than other quality assurance data; and (4) data from consumers provide information not available from any other source (Davies and Ware 1988).

Consumers' behavior can often be predicted by their quality assessments. Thus, complaints, switching doctors, disenrollment, compliance with treatment and utilization have been linked by various studies to consumer attitudes about the quality of providers (Ware et al. 1981; Mirowsky and Ross 1983).

Consumers' reports of what happened during medical care encounters tend to be accurate. Ware et al. (1978) found that the overall accuracy of patients' recall of what happened during a visit to the physician tended to be very high. Likewise, Gerbert and Hargreaves (1987) found patient and physicians agreed 96 percent of the time in recalling tests ordered, 94 percent for treatments mentioned, and 88 percent on occurrence of patient education. These results indicate that consumers' reports hold considerable potential as a data source for quality assurance programs (Davies and Ware 1988). Compared to expert review or audit of medical records, consumer survey data are no more expensive and in many cases less expensive than obtaining data in the traditional way (Davies and Ware 1988).

Finally, a major reason for using consumer surveys is that they provide information unavailable from any other source. It is particularly difficult to use traditional quality assurance methods and databases for outpatient care. Outpatient records are often difficult to obtain from office-based physicians, and they may be incomplete particularly with respect to recording negative findings (Davies and Ware 1988). Consumer surveys, however, can be used effectively to evaluate both inpatient and outpatient care.

While many quality assurance measures focus on the technical nature of medical care or the quantity of care, they may overlook the interpersonal nature of such care or the communication between doctor and patient. Consumer surveys may be the best instruments for measuring this "art of care" or the "humaneness" dimension of quality care.

We should remember that most consumer surveys weight questions equally, when in the consumer's mind not all elements of health care may have the same value. For example, HMO consumers might rate access to care, availability of care and other dimensions of care rather poorly yet still remain in the HMO because they are most concerned about costs. HMOs achieve cost reductions by reducing some amenities available in FFS settings. For many HMO members, cost may be the most important variable. Once in the HMO, however, other factors, such as waiting time, become more important (Luft 1981).

Finally, we should keep in mind that HMO members are a self-selected group that tend to be better informed and more active than the general population (Luft 1981). Therefore, they may be more inclined to be critical of their health care when it fails to meet their higher expectations. If all consumers were as informed and active as HMO members, their expectations of FFS providers could also be higher, and thus their evaluations might be lower.

## COMPARISONS OF CONSUMERS' SATISFACTION

Most studies of consumer satisfaction of health care concern issues of access to care, continuity of care, technical quality, humaneness, cost, and overall satisfaction. These are discussed below.

### Access to Care

Since HMOs contain costs at least in part by restricting access, particularly access to specialists and hospitals, one would expect that most HMO enrollees would be less satisfied with access than their FFS counterparts. Yet, most comparative surveys on access by HMO and FFS enrollees provide only partial support for this assumption. Indeed, the most striking factor is the comparatively small difference in perceived access between HMO and FFS patients (Luft 1981).

The two most often used measures of access are the time one waits to obtain an appointment with a doctor and the time one waits in the doctor's office. HMO patients typically wait longer than FFS patients for an appointment, but they wait less in the office. HMOs, particularly staff and group-models, attempt to

**Table 4.1**
**Comparison of HMO Members and Eligible Nonmembers Satisfaction with Access to Health Care**

| | HMO Members | Eligible Nonmembers |
|---|---|---|
| Ability to See a Doctor Whenever Needed | | |
| Very Satisfied | 55% | 38% |
| Somewhat Satisfied | 31% | 40% |
| Very/Somewhat Dissatisfied | 13% | 20% |
| The Availability of Doctors and Medical Services 24 Hours A Day, 7 Days A Week | | |
| Very Satisfied | 49% | 32% |
| Somewhat Satisfied | 32% | 34% |
| Very/Somewhat Dissatisfied | 16% | 33% |
| The Amount of Time You Have to Wait to See a Doctor After You Have Called For An Appointment | | |
| Very Satisfied | 31% | 25% |
| Somewhat Satisfied | 38% | 34% |
| Very/Somewhat Dissatisfied | 32% | 40% |
| Ability to See a Specialist When You Need One | | |
| Very Satisfied | 48% | 42% |
| Somewhat Satisfied | 29% | 42% |
| Very/Somewhat Dissatisfied | 15% | 13% |

*Source*: Louis Harris and Associates. *A Report Card on HMOs: Summary Report*, 1984. Reprinted with permission.

keep their physicians fully occupied by maintaining full-time appointment schedules. On the other hand, the FFS doctor maintains a more flexible schedule and ''squeezes'' patients into the schedule. Indeed, the FFS doctor may often overbook in order to maximize income and to compensate for possible ''no-shows.''

Most satisfaction surveys reveal that HMO enrollees are satisfied with access. Davies et al. (1986) found that HMO enrollees rated office waits significantly more favorably, while the FFS group had significantly more favorable attitudes toward appointment waits. Wagner and Bledsoe (1990) found the same. Murray (1987) found no significant difference among HMO and FFS patients in their rating of access to care. A Harris survey (Table 4.1) found that 55 percent of HMO members were very satisfied with their ability to see a doctor whenever needed compared to only 38 percent of non-HMO consumers. Likewise, more HMO members were satisfied with the availability of doctors and specialists and with the amount of time that one had to wait to see a doctor.

A 1989 survey revealed that nine out of ten HMO members who had received routine care in the past year were satisfied with the waiting time between making an appointment and seeing their doctor (Blue Cross and Blue Shield 1989). The average waiting time for a routine appointment was approximately one week. The same survey revealed that 83 percent of the respondents were satisfied with the amount of time they had to sit in the waiting room before seeing their doctor, which averaged about twenty minutes.

Clearly, HMOs do not appear to significantly reduce access even as they curtail utilization. Indeed, PGPs enjoy a clear advantage in shorter office waiting times (Luft 1981). This may be balanced by waiting longer to obtain an appointment. For routine health care problems, PGPs pose no access problems. For those with nonroutine problems who may need a specialist, they may have to wait somewhat longer than the average FFS patient (Davies et al. 1986).

### Continuity of Care

After receiving basic access to care, patients may seek continuity of care. Most believe it is a significant factor in the total quality of care. Yet, there may be different definitions of continuity of care. Does it mean care from the same doctor, or the same group, or in the same physical location? Most probably define it as care from the same doctor.

Murray (1987) found no significant differences in HMO and FFS patients' satisfaction with continuity of care. However, Davies et al. (1986) found that FFS consumers were significantly more satisfied with continuity of care. Other studies yield mixed results. Many who join an HMO must break ties with their FFS providers. Thus, they are predisposed to perceive greater discontinuity even when they are seeing the same HMO doctor at each visit. This may be particularly the case in PGPs where there is a more limited choice of physicians and where past FFS ties must be broken.

When discontinuity is measured by the identification of a single physician, PGPs may provide less continuity of care. On the other hand, PGPs may be better able to maintain continuity of medical record transfers in more serious cases when specialists are required or hospitalization is needed.

### Technical Competence

The Harris survey (1984) found 50 percent of HMO members were very satisfied with the quality of their doctors and another 40 percent were somewhat satisfied. In comparison, 47 percent of non-HMO members were very satisfied and another 38 percent somewhat satisfied. Similarly, 57 percent of the HMO members were very satisfied with the quality of their hospital care compared to 34 percent of nonmembers who were very satisfied. Only 9 percent of the HMO members were very or somewhat dissatisfied compared to 19 percent of the non-HMO members.

Davies et al. (1986) found no difference in satisfaction with the technical quality of care between average HMO and FFS members. However, they did find that the higher-income sick HMO members who had been accustomed to buying the amount of care they wanted in the FFS system, tended to be disappointed with the technical quality of care in HMOs. Davies et al. (1986) conclude that this less favorable rating of technical competence by the higher income group reflected their equating less care with less thorough care. From these studies, it appears that consumers believe HMOs generally offer care that is technically competent. At least, there is no clear, consistent pattern that HMO members are dissatisfied with the technical quality of their health care.

**Humanness**

Patients are often just as concerned about their doctors' "bedside manners" as they are about their technical competence. By "bedside manners," we often mean the degree to which doctors and other providers are friendly, caring, compassionate, empathetic, and communicative. In a review of several studies, Luft (1981) found PGP enrollees were often less satisfied with their physicians' willingness to listen and to explain. On the other hand, Davies et al. (1986) found no significant differences between the satisfaction of HMO members and nonmembers with their doctors' answers to questions.

Luft (1981) also found that PGP enrollees were generally less satisfied than FFS consumers with their doctors' friendliness, warmth, and personal interest. While Murray (1987) found no significant differences in the humanness variables among the FFS and HMO members, Davies et al. (1986) found that the FFS patients tended to rate their doctors higher on these variables.

The mixed opinions of HMO enrollees toward the interpersonal aspects of their care may be traced to the possibility of less continuity of care by personal physicians in HMOs. This is more possible in PGPs than in IPAs. Of course, such discontinuity can interfere with the development of doctor-patient relationships.

Davies et al. (1986) found that HMO members' dissatisfaction with the interpersonal aspects of their care was greatest when they first enrolled in an HMO and subsided after three to five years experience in the HMO. When joining an HMO, discontinuity in medical care providers may be most pronounced for the new HMO members. However, as the discontinuity subsides, and as the new members gain experience with the HMO doctors, their dissatisfaction also subsides.

The lower satisfaction of HMO enrollees with the humanness of doctors may also be a product of the tight scheduling of appointments in PGPs. While such scheduling means less waiting time in the doctor's office, it also means that the doctor has only a set amount of time to spend with each patient. Thus, the doctor may not take more time to explain procedures, ask questions and generally interact with the patient. Of course, the patient may view this strict adherence to schedule as cold, uncaring, uncommunicative behavior.

### Costs of Care

Most consumers probably join HMOs because of the costs and coverage provided by HMOs. Satisfaction studies tend to confirm that HMO members are significantly more satisfied with the costs of health care than are FFS consumers. Luft's extensive review (1981) found that HMO members were consistently more satisfied with the costs and coverage provided by HMOs.

A Louis Harris survey reveals that HMO members are much more satisfied with their benefits and the costs of their health care (see Table 4.2). Likewise, Murray (1987) found that HMO members were significantly more satisfied with the costs of their health plan. Davis et al. (1986) found the same. A 1989 survey revealed that what most HMO members liked most about their health plan was the cost and benefit coverage (Blue Cross and Blue Shield 1989). These studies clearly reveal that HMO members are more satisfied than the average FFS patient with their health care benefits and the cost of these benefits.

### Overall Satisfaction

Comparisons of the overall satisfaction of HMO members and nonmembers with their health plans show mixed results. Some research indicates that HMO members are more generally satisfied (Louis Harris and Associates 1984). Yet, others show no significant difference in overall satisfaction (Murray 1987). Still others show that FFS consumers are significantly more satisfied overall (Davies et al. 1986).

## DISENROLLMENT AS A SIGN OF CONSUMER DISSATISFACTION

A behavioral indicator of consumer dissatisfaction with quality could be the decision to leave an HMO. However, all disenrollments do not reflect dissatisfaction. Much disenrollment is involuntary. When employees change or lose their jobs, they may not be covered by the same HMO. Therefore, they would probably disenroll. Such involuntary disenrollment does not necessarily reflect dissatisfaction. On the other hand, voluntary decisions to disenroll generally reflect some dissatisfaction.

Most studies of disenrollment reveal that only a small percentage (7 to 14 percent) of HMO members voluntarily disenroll annually (Luft 1981, Lewis 1984). Of course, such disenrollment could reflect dissatisfaction with costs or quality, and the limited literature provides no conclusive answer. Moreover, it is not clear how these relatively small percentages compare to disenrollment

**Table 4.2**
**Comparison of HMO Members and Eligible Nonmembers Satisfaction with Health Plan Benefits**

| | HMO Members | Eligible Nonmembers |
|---|---|---|
| How Much of Your Family's Major Medical Expenses for Surgery and Serious Illness Are Paid For | | |
| Very Satisfied | 72% | 47% |
| Somewhat Satisfied | 19% | 36% |
| Very/Somewhat Dissatisfied | 5% | 13% |
| How Much You and Your Family Pay Compared to What the Insurance or Plan Pays | | |
| Very Satisfied | 68% | 41% |
| Somewhat Satisfied | 21% | 40% |
| Very/Somewhat Dissatisfied | 8% | 16% |
| The Cost of Your Health Plan's Premiums | | |
| Very Satisfied | 57% | 48% |
| Somewhat Satisfied | 29% | 30% |
| Very/Somewhat Dissatisfied | 13% | 18% |
| How Much of Your Family Treatments for Minor Illness and Lab Tests Are Paid For | | |
| Very Satisfied | 74% | 35% |
| Somewhat Satisfied | 19% | 35% |
| Very/Somewhat Dissatisfied | 6% | 28% |
| How Much of Your Family's Doctors' Visits Are Paid For | | |
| Very Satisfied | 72% | 35% |
| Somewhat Satisfied | 20% | 38% |
| Very/Somewhat Dissatisfied | 7% | 23% |

*Source*: Louis Harris and Associates. *A Report Card on HMOs: Summary Report*, 1984. Reprinted with permission.

from fee-for-service arrangements. Indeed, it is difficult to conceptualize or define disenrollment from the fee-for-service system. Would movement from one fee-for-service provider to another fee-for-service provider constitute disenrollment? Or would a consumer have to completely abandon fee-for-service arrangements before they could be considered disenrollees? Of course, there must be an HMO option available in a community before one can completely abandon fee-for-service providers.

The choice of moving from an HMO to a fee-for-service plan is not symmetrical with the choice of moving from a fee-for-service plan to an HMO (Luft 1981). Consumers have experience with fee-for-service arrangements, but often know very little about HMOs. Thus, if consumers are hesitant to use what they do not know, then they will be more likely to switch from HMOs to fee-for-service than the converse.

The low rates of voluntary disenrollments from HMOs and the difficulty in determining whether cost or quality considerations caused the disenrollments, plus the lack of solid comparative data for traditional indemnity programs, indicate that consumer dissatisfaction with the quality of care in HMOs is not great.

## SUMMARY OF SATISFACTION STUDIES

Given HMOs' strong incentive to control costs by reducing utilization, it is surprising that HMO members do not have more negative attitudes toward HMOs. Considering that HMOs often have longer waiting times to get an appointment and shorter average time with the doctor, one might expect even more dissatisfaction. Yet, in general most HMO members are satisfied with their plans. They are particularly satisfied with their plans' costs and benefits. HMO members are generally as satisfied as FFS patients with the access and availability of care. However, they may have some concern about access to a specialist. Similarly, they may have greater concerns about continuity of care.

FFS and HMO patients are equally satisfied with the technical competence of their doctors. However, more HMO members than FFS patients may be concerned about their doctors' warmth and interpersonal relations.

## QUALITY AND ACCREDITATION OF HMOs

Several organizations seek to validate or assure minimal levels of quality through their accreditation of HMOs. The three major national accreditation organizations that are currently accreditating HMOs are (1) the Joint Commission on the Accreditation of Healthcare Organizations (JCAHO), (2) the National Committee for Quality Assurance (NCQA), and (3) the Accreditation Association for Ambulatory Health Care (AAAHC).

JCAHO was established by a group of hospitals and medical associations in 1951 for the purpose of accreditation of hospitals. Later, it began accrediting a wide range of health care organizations such as outpatient centers, group practices, community health centers, hospices, home care organizations, nursing homes, and substance abuse programs (Joint Commission 1989). Thus, it was only natural for JCAHO to move into the accreditation of HMOs in the mid-1980s.

In 1985, JCAHO responded to a request to define standards and conduct quality surveys of 11 HMOs in Ohio that contracted to provide care to Medicaid patients. Likewise, JCAHO has done the same for Medicaid contracting HMOs in South Carolina and Minnesota. Also, it has conducted reviews for HMOs of the Prudential Insurance Company. In 1988, it signed an initial agreement to become the official accreditation agency for 96 percent of the HMOs operating under the Blue Cross/Blue Shield umbrella.

The National Committee for Quality Assurance (NCQA) was formed in 1979 as a joint venture between the Group Health Association of America (GHAA) and the American Medical Care and Review Association (AMCRA) to help HMOs and group practices develop and operate quality assurance programs. Its original purpose was to conduct quality reviews for the Office of Health Maintenance Organizations (OHMO) of the U.S. Department of Health and Human Services as part of the federal qualification process (National Committee for Quality Assurance 1990). Thus, it completed over 60 reviews of HMOs in Pennsylvania as part of the federal qualification and state licensure process. Subsequently, it was less active due to budget cutbacks that precluded OHMO from continuing to contract for quality reviews.

In 1987, it became clear that NCQA needed a greater degree of independence to assure its independence from the HMO industry while maintaining strong HMO input. Thus, the board was reconstituted as a self-perpetuating body representing HMOs, employers, unions, and consumers. NCQA is exclusively concerned with health maintenance organizations and does not review hospitals or other types of providers, nor does it review ambulatory organizations in the fee-for-service sector.

Currently, NCQA is reviewing HMOs for licensure purposes in Pennsylvania and Kansas. In Michigan, NCQA is coordinating efforts of the state, the three automobile companies, and the United Auto Workers directed at the development and implementation of a quality review process.

Like JCAHO, the Accreditation Association for Ambulatory Health Care (AAAHC) was organized by a group of healthcare organizations but concentrated on ambulatory care. It has accredited almost 200 group practices, including some affiliated with HMOs. During the last two years, the AAAHC has become more involved in reviewing HMOs and has accredited forty-seven CIGNA plans. It has also contracted with Arizona and Hawaii to review the quality of HMO services provided to Medicaid patients.

All three accrediting bodies have core standards that emphasize the development of quality assurance programs in HMOs and the maintenance of comprehensive medical records and information systems. All accreditation reviews involve an assessment of an HMO's overall structure, its quality assurance program, provider credentials, utilization data, grievance procedures, and risk sharing arrangements.

While these three accrediting bodies have accredited over 200 HMOs, many HMOs remain unaccredited. Although it seems reasonable to assume that accredited HMOs provide higher quality care than nonaccredited HMOs, there is little research on this comparison. Accreditation by definition emphasizes the structural and process dimensions of quality. Whether these structural and process advantages provide better outcomes in HMOs remains unclear.

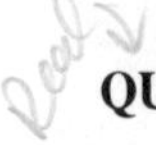

## QUALITY ASSURANCE IN HMOs

Employers are increasingly concerned about the quality of care their employees receive from HMOs. Some worry that cost containment is purchased at the expense of quality. Others are concerned about being liable when their employees receive inadequate health care. Thus, employers are growing increasingly interested in HMOs' quality assurance processes.

There are a number of basic components in an effective quality assurance (QA) process that employers should review when contracting with an HMO. First, quality care is impossible without well-qualified providers. Any HMO should have a standardized, rigorous process for reviewing physicians and others providers' license to practice and their training, references, and board certification. Considering that a 1986 study found that 50 percent of physicians applying for clinical positions in a national ambulatory care program presented false clinical credentials, the HMO review process is even more important (Schaffer et al. 1988).

In network, group, and IPA HMOs, the physician group and individual physician offices and facilities as well as their medical records system, safety procedures, and administrative structure should be reviewed prior to the issuance of contracts.

Reappointment of providers is as important as their initial appointment. HMOs should have a standard periodic review of a physician's past history in the HMO including utilization data, patient complaints, and complications.

Employers should inquire about an HMO's continuing medical education program. Also, information concerning the ratio of staff to patients by professional category should be obtained. In addition, the employer should ask the HMO how it utilizes the services of nonphysicians (e.g., registered nurses, physician assistants and nurse practitioners) and under what circumstances.

Employers should also ask if the HMO has QA contracts with physicians which the physicians accept when they enter the HMO. Likewise, employers should ask to see the HMO's QA contracts with major providers such as hospitals and pharmacies. These contracts should detail the QA activities that the contracting institution agrees to perform (Joint Commission 1989). The employer might also inquire into the range of services offered by the HMO's hospital as well as its age/sex case mix adjusted mortality rates.

After reviewing how an HMO appoints and reappoints its providers, the employer should ask to see the HMO's QA plan. If an HMO is seriously concerned about quality, it should have a written plan that has high visibility throughout the organization. The plan should delineate its goals, scope of activities, monitoring and reporting mechanisms, the practitioner's role in the QA process, and the authority and responsibility relationships among those charged with QA, the providers, and the HMO's administrators.

The plan should clearly state that a QA committee or an individual (often the medical director) is responsible for the QA process. This group or individual should (1) be accountable to the CEO of the HMO or the governing board, (2) prepare at least annual QA reports that are reviewed by the HMO's board, (3) hold regularly scheduled meetings or activities specifically focused on measuring quality, and (4) maintain records of QA recommendations and actions (National Committee for Quality Assurance 1990).

The more visible the QA committee or position is in the HMO, the more effective it is likely to be. If it has access to operating management meetings and to all data bases, including files of malpractice claims, member complaints, surveys, utilization data, medical records, and claims data, it is much more likely to be a positive force for quality (Berwick 1987).

The QA committee or leader should review the scope of care provided by the HMO in order to identify the important aspects of care. These are cases or areas of care that occur frequently and which affect many or which have caused problems in the past. Once these important areas of care have been identified, the QA leaders should select indicators of the quality of care in each area. For example, indicators of care in cancer screening could include participation rates in screening, stool blood testing annually for individuals over forty years of age, and yearly mammography for women over fifty years of age (Joint Commission 1989).

Indicators are used to identify problems that HMOs should address. Other methods to recognize problems are patient surveys. Such surveys can reveal the members' perception of quality. Patients are particularly capable of judging access to care and the humanness and sensitivity of providers.

Other methods of identifying patient dissatisfaction are the rates of voluntary disenrollment and the number of malpractice suits. Employers should ask to see summaries of these surveys. Another way of judging patient dissatisfaction is to review the grievance process in the HMO. Employers should ask to see summaries of member grievances and their disposition.

Documenting the level of quality is impossible without a sound management information system in an HMO. HMOs should have well-developed systems for the collection, retrieval and distribution of patient records. Moreover, there should be one position responsible for the confidentiality and security of such records. Particular attention must be given to records management in open-panel IPAs that contract with many independent physicians who have their own unique record systems. It is particularly difficult in such situations to monitor continuity of care as the patient moves from one provider to another.

After the QA process identifies problems, it should issue recommendations to solve them. Thus, an employer should ask the HMO for a summary of all recommendations developed by the QA process over the last year or two and for a brief description of the HMO's actions in pursuit of the recommendations. Answers to these questions can indicate whether the HMO's QA process actually identifies problems that lead to recommendations, and whether such recommendations are taken seriously by the HMO's leaders.

According to Berwick (1987), there are two major threats to quality in HMOs. One is inadequate access to care. Thus, the QA process in an HMO should give particular attention to the timing of scheduled appointments. Since waiting lists are the primary way in which HMOs ration care, employers should be particularly concerned about the waiting time to schedule an appointment. It should not exceed two or two and a half weeks (Meier and Aquilina 1982). Likewise, employers should ask about the average waiting time in a doctor's office. It should not exceed 15 to 30 minutes (Meier and Aquilina 1982).

The second threat is failure to integrate care. HMOs structure often requires the transfer of patients across many lines. Therefore, the safety and comfort of the patient require secure forms of communication and coordination (Berwick 1987). HMOs should have procedures to ensure that any enrollee has a personal physician who coordinates all of the enrollee's medical care. Every enrollee should be offered assistance in selecting a personal physician and should be allowed to switch if dissatisfied.

## CONCLUSION

While the field of quality assessment in health care is not as advanced as one would like, the available measures indicate that HMOs provide quality care equal to if not better than that provided by fee-for-service providers. HMOs seem particularly suited to score well on structural dimensions of care. HMOs, particularly staff and group-model HMOs, have formal organizational structures that tend to promote more comprehensive and better integrated care than that provided by solo, fee-for-service practitioners. Also, the credentials and performance of providers in HMOs are more likely to be reviewed periodically than are those of solo practitioners.

HMOs tend to emphasize continuing education for their providers. Likewise, most HMOs have internal quality assurance and peer review processes that promote quality care. These are generally less available among solo practitioners in fee-for-service settings. Thus, it should not be too surprising that most studies indicate HMOs deliver care at least equal to that found in the fee-for-service sector.

The favorable evidence of HMOs' performance on structural, process, and outcome measures of quality is generally supported by satisfaction surveys of HMO members. Most surveys show enrollees are satisfied with their access to care and the technical competence of their providers. The major areas of concern for HMO members are continuity of care and the humanness of their providers. Both of these concerns may be explained by the necessity for the new HMO enrollee to change doctors when they join an HMO. Thus, they may be predisposed to perceive greater discontinuity even when they see the same HMO doctor during each visit.

The HMO enrollees' satisfaction with care seems particularly impressive when one considers that HMOs have strong economic incentives to limit costs by restricting access. Likewise, HMO doctors have similar incentives not to spend very much time with each patient. Moreover, HMOs achieve cost reductions by reducing some amenities available in the FFS sector. Cost may be the most important reason why many join an HMO. But once in the HMO, enrollees may complain about the very things that produced the lower costs. Finally, we should remember that HMO members are self-selected individuals who probably are better informed than the average consumer, and thus may be more likely to be critical of their health care when it fails to meet their higher expectations. Given all these handicaps, HMOs are rated surprisingly well by their members.

Since HMOs have obvious economic incentives to practice conservative medicine or follow a "wait and see" strategy rather than an aggressive diagnostic strategy, some patients' problems will not be properly diagnosed at an early stage, and they will not be referred to a specialist or admitted to a hospital at the appropriate time. While the total effect of this conservative strategy does not appear to affect HMOs' overall health outcomes, it is detrimental to the early detection and treatment of some cases.

The conservative strategy may become more detrimental to health care quality as competition becomes more intense among HMOs, as the number of physicians increase, and as the number of private, investor owned HMOs increase. All of these factors place even more pressure on physicians to guard the economic bottom line by pursuing an even more conservative approach to medicine.

Likewise, the dramatic growth in IPA-type HMOs, and the increasing tendency for HMOs to contract with individual solo practitioners may have negative impacts on quality. Most of the quality studies that compare care in HMO and FFS settings have reviewed staff or group-model HMOs, not IPAs. In general, most staff and group-model HMOs have more formal structures for quality control and peer reviews than do IPAs. It is inevitably more difficult to control quality in the multiple, geographically dispersed doctors' offices of IPAs. The monitoring of medical record data is much more difficult.

As risk pools of HMOs are reduced to include fewer and fewer physicians, the economic incentives for each physician to provide less care becomes more and more persuasive. Indeed, more and more IPAs contract with individual physicians on a capitated basis, and the individual physician is at risk for all costs above the capitated amount. Of course, such arrangements contain obvious threats to quality.

These concerns about recent developments in HMOs highlight the absolute necessity for effective quality assurance processes in HMOs, particularly in IPAs. Employers who are concerned about the health of their employees and who seek quality medical care for their health care dollar, should demand that HMOs document their efforts to monitor and assure quality health care.

# 5

# HMOs and Employers

Over the past several years, there has been increasing tension between HMOs and employers. This can be seen in changing employer attitudes about HMOs' ability to control costs. A 1986 national survey (Johnson and Higgins 1986) found that only 14 percent of employers disagreed with the statement that "HMOs are effective in controlling costs." However, by 1987, 22 percent disagreed with the statement (Foster Higgins 1987), and in 1988, over 32 percent disagreed (Foster Higgins 1988). Thus, more and more employers are becoming disenchanted with HMOs.

Much of employers' discomfort can be traced to provisions of the HMO Act of 1973. Specifically, employers found fault with the (1) dual choice mandate, (2) the mandated rating requirements, (3) the equal dollar contribution requirement, (4) the federal qualification process, and (5) the insufficient data requirements of the law.

## DUAL-CHOICE MANDATE

The 1973 HMO Act allowed federally qualified HMOs to mandate that employers with twenty-five or more employees offer at least one staff or group-model and one IPA or direct contract model HMO provided that they were available in the area. Of course, the original motive behind this provision of the law was to provide HMOs access to commercial markets in areas where employers opposed HMOs.

While there may have been a need for the dual-choice mandate in 1973, most employers believe there is no longer a need for it. Conditions have changed since 1973. HMOs are accepted much more readily in most areas of the country, and membership in HMOs has escalated dramatically (Peres 1988). Thus, the necessity of mandating appears weak. Indeed, perhaps 80 to 90 percent of all HMO/employer contracts are voluntary and did not result from the mandating process (Wrightson 1990).

In an increasingly competitive health care environment, the mandate may not be particularly good for HMOs or employers. First, it casts a negative tone over relations between employers and HMOs (Peres 1988). Thus, employers could respond to a mandate in a manner that could delay its implementation or stop it completely. For example, they could raise numerous technical objections and increase delays. They could select an alternative federally qualified HMO rather than the plan that initiated the mandate. Moreover, they could establish a pattern of employer contributions that would lead to adverse selection into the HMO or create an environment that could minimize the HMO's enrollment of eligible employees. In addition, the employer could drop a mandating HMO as soon as possible since the 1973 Act is unclear on the length of time that a particular HMO mandate is valid (Peres 1988).

## HMO ACT RATING REQUIREMENTS

Employers have opposed the 1973 HMO Act's requirement that federally mandated HMOs must use community rating. In order to understand the nature of this opposition one must have a basic understanding of rating and the different types of rating.

### Rating

To rate is to determine or set the amount of the premium or money charged to provide a specific unit of insurance for a particular group. There are often competing goals and criteria for evaluating a rating system. For example, rating systems must satisfy the conflicting objectives of management, policyholders, marketing personnel, and stockholders, if it is a for-profit organization (Wrightson 1990). Policyholders will want the system to generate just enough money to cover expenses. Conversely, shareholders want a system that will generate maximum profits. Likewise, management seeks a system that will permit growth in sales, maximize profits, minimize costs, and maintain the morale of the sales force. The marketing personnel are primarily interested in maximizing sales through competitive rates. Obviously, all of these goals cannot be maximized simultaneously.

Any rating system must be (1) efficient, that is, generate revenue sufficient to cover expenses, (2) competitive, (3) equitable, (4) simple, (5) flexible, and (6) consistent (Wrightson 1990). Of these qualities, the most difficult to define or achieve may be equity, which refers to the perceived fairness of the premium rates (Wrightson 1990).

Rates for group health insurance may reasonably vary based on a number of factors including health care benefits provided, demographic nature of the group, prior claims experience of the group, and other characteristics of the group such as size, industry, and geographic location. Many believe that "equity" indicates self-supporting premiums or rates. Accordingly, the rates charged to a group would be equal to the money needed to offset the expected costs of the group. While this seems logical at first glance, if it is followed in the extreme, the basic goal of insurance (pooling of risks) would be endangered. As a result, every group, however small, would be self-insured. Thus, equity generally implies that self-supporting premiums are applied to classes of groups in order to provide a sufficiently large group to pool risks successfully (Wrightson 1990).

### Community Rating

Community rating bases premiums on the costs of the entire community of individuals in an HMO. It does not attempt, like experience rating, to base rates on the actual health care experience of a particular group. In community rating, planwide costs are projected for the next year and the total costs are divided equally among all members of the plan (Sutton 1986). Thus, the same premium rates are offered to all employers regardless of the health care experience of any specific employer's employees. Riders may be added for additional benefits such as prescriptions, dental, and vision care. These riders are also community-rated so that all employees who select the rider pay the same rate.

Community rating has been used overwhelmingly by HMOs for a variety of reasons. Community rating was used by the first prepaid group plans such as Kaiser Permanente and so became part of the original cost-containment philosophy of prepaid groups (Sutton 1986). Some believed that if HMOs based rates on actual "experience" or actual service, the rating system would continue to encourage traditional fee-for-service medicine and thus be antithetical to the underlying HMO philosophy and incentives.

Compared to other rating systems, community rating is relatively simple. HMOs using this system do not need large underwriting units to determine premium increases for many different employer groups. The data requirements and management information systems are much less elaborate. As a result, these HMO overhead expenses are considerably reduced.

Community rating results in revenue projections that are much more stable and predictable than those resulting from other rating systems. Predictability of revenues is a major need of HMOs, particularly staff and group-model HMOs, which may have considerable fixed costs in capital facilities (hospitals, clinics, computers, and so on) and salaried personnel (physicians, technicians, nurses, administrative personnel).

Community rating also produces more stable rates since the premiums are based on the experience of the entire population of the HMO. Conversely, rates based on the experience of each employer group are much more likely to be less stable and large year-to-year fluctuations in premium increases could result. Since most HMOs are part of multiple option programs offered by employers, any single HMO rarely enrolls all of a company's employees. Thus, many HMOs are composed of many relatively small employee groups. Therefore, the volatility of rate increases could be considerable if rates were based on the actual experience of the small group (Sutton 1986).

Many believe that community rating is fairer and more equitable than experience rating. Since community rating spreads costs over the entire enrollment rather than basing premiums on enrollees' age, sex, and health status, it more effectively pools risks, which is an underlying philosophy of prepaid plans.

Over time community rating has become very traditional within most HMOs. Hence, any new system would be quite disruptive in many HMOs, particularly group and staff models which use community rating overwhelmingly.

Community rating requires that HMOs have data on inpatient utilization rates, hospital costs, frequency of visits to physician offices, physician costs, number and costs of ancillary services (X rays, laboratory tests, prescriptions), other demographic data (sex and age of HMO populations), and administrative costs (personnel salary, marketing, data processing, supplies, telephones).

The actual process of using this information to determine rates is often a function of the HMO's form and structure (Wrightson 1990). Most staff-model HMOs and some group HMOs build their projected revenue requirement by a budgeting approach. In contrast, IPAs and network type HMOs often use an actuarial approach to develop a capitation rate.

Under the budgeting approach, a budget forecast and enrollment predictions are used to determine premium rate increases. The budget forecast is based on recent historical costs for the data items noted above adjusted to reflect inflation and enrollment changes. Likewise, revenue projections are based on recent revenue receipts from premiums, copayments, third-party payments, reinsurance payments, fee-for-service and interest. These are adjusted to reflect projected enrollment changes. The projected revenues and expenses are compared, and any shortfall becomes the premium rate increase. Since most HMOs have low levels of surplus capital, it is critical that the revenue and expenditure projections be accurate.

In contrast to the budgeting approach used by most staff-model HMOs, most IPA and network type HMOs use an actuarial approach to develop a capitation rate on a service-by-service basis. This method projects the costs per member per month by projecting the utilization rate of each service and the unit cost of the service (Wrightson 1990).

Whether an HMO uses the budgeting or actuarial approach to determine premium rate increases, other factors such as profit orientation, federal qualification status, and plan sponsorship can also affect rates. For example, profit HMOs must produce profits for its stockholders, and thus they are under greater pressure to increase rates. A federally-qualified HMO must offer a set of comprehensive benefits and therefore cannot offer a very low-cost option. A plan sponsored by physicians will have different approaches to physician reimbursement and risk-sharing policies than an HMO sponsored by an insurance company (Wrightson

1990). Likewise, the selection of providers by an HMO can affect rates. An HMO that seeks the highest quality and thus contracts with university hospital and medical centers will have different rates than an HMO that contracts with community hospitals.

### Experience Rating

Unlike community rating, which bases premiums on the average cost of all enrollees in a plan, experience rating bases rates on the actual health expenditures of a specific group. Under experience rating, for example, a particular employer might pay a premium based on the actual health care costs of the company's employees. Private insurers have used experience rating for many decades to determine premiums for large organizations. Experience rating requires considerably more data than does community rating. Costs for hospitals, physicians, ancillary services as well as costs involving marketing, administration, and claims processing must be allocated to specific employer groups. Moreover, since premiums are based on actual costs, HMOs using experience rating must be much more concerned about reporting mechanisms because they often have to provide detailed reports documenting the services used by a particular employer group. Likewise, HMOs using experience rating must be much more proficient in evaluating the characteristics of groups which could affect utilization of health care (e.g., age, sex composition, health care history, industry and any other factor that could affect costs).

Basically, there are two forms of experience rating: retrospective and prospective. Under prospective rating, the recent historical costs are used to predict future costs and premiums. If the actual costs are higher than the predicted costs, the HMO must "eat" the loss. On the other hand, if the actual costs are less than the predicted costs, the HMO may pocket the surplus.

Retrospective rating also uses historical cost data to project future rates. However, if the premiums generate more income than the actual costs, a refund is made to the employer, or the refund is placed in a reserve fund and used to balance future shortages, or a refund may be returned to the employer in the form of a credit against future premiums. When the actual costs are greater than the premiums, the employer may be required to pay more, or payments may be withdrawn from the reserve fund, or future premiums may reflect the loss.

### Problems of Community Rating

Employers generally are uncomfortable with community rating (Luft 1985b). Most believe that they would like to pay for only the health care costs of their employees. Employers are often suspicious of community rating and believe that they are subsidizing another employer's employees. Obviously, some cross-subsidizing does occur under community rating. Some low-risk groups subsidize some high-risk groups. This is inherent in the basic philosophy behind the approach. However, most employers overlook the fact that they could benefit as well as lose from cross subsidies. They generally perceive the losses, but not the benefits. In any case, most employers, particularly the larger employers, want to pay for only what they use. In short, they want experience rating.

As noted in the earlier section on favorable selection bias into HMOs, many employers believe that HMOs "skim" their employee population and enroll the healthier, lower-risk individuals. They also suspect that the actual health care costs of these healthier employees are lower than the community rates charged by HMOs. Employers often believe that HMOs use many of the specific practices noted in Chapter 3 (providing well-baby coverage, preventive dentistry, and sports medicine to attract younger, low-risk employees) to encourage the healthy to enroll and to discourage enrollment by the high-risk group.

Thus employers often conclude that as HMOs attract the healthier employees, the remaining higher-risk employees in the traditional indemnity plans generate higher premiums. As the premiums, deductibles, and co-payments increase for the remaining higher-risk pool, the healthier employees within this pool continue to seek the lower cost alternatives of HMOs. Thus, the indemnity insurance plan grows increasingly more expensive for employers.

Employers often do not see much face validity in HMOs' rate setting process (Wrightson 1990). Some employers assert that HMOs do not give the same rate to all groups for the same level of benefits even though community rating implies equal rates. They complain that some HMOs cannot document or explain how they derived their community rates.

Similarly, some employers claim that HMOs often "shadow price" their rates just below those charged by traditional indemnity insurers. According to employers, if HMOs attract the healthier employees, leaving the costlier employees in the indemnity plans, then the community rates should be significantly below the premiums charged by the indemnity plans. But, employers insist that this is often not the case and that the HMO rates are often just below the indemnity rates, resulting in windfall profits for HMOs.

Of course, HMOs claim that these criticisms are overstated. First, they insist that they do not have a population of healthier enrollees. Second, if they save money, it is because of their cost-containment efforts, not the result of biased selection. Third, they plead that they do offer the community rates and do not shadow price. Unfortunately, many HMOs do not gather sufficient data to document their cost experience with any particular employer group. As a result, they are not well positioned to justify or explain their rates.

Because of the increasingly competitive market in managed health care, many HMOs are beginning to rethink their traditional adherence to community rating. In a very competitive market, many of the touted advantages of community rating tend to disappear (Wrightson 1990). If aggressive indemnity plans offer low premiums to low-cost groups, then an HMO will experience serious adverse disenrollment and loss of revenues. Historically, community-rated health plans have suffered when they encountered vigorous competition from experience-rated plans. For example, Blue Cross plans were originally community rated, but subsequently moved to experience rating as a result of competition (Sutton 1986).

As long as HMOs community rate, they may not be in a good position to estimate the likely costs of a particular employee group. On the other hand, traditional indemnity plans with large underwriting departments may be able to generate the statistical analyses necessary for accurate prediction of costs. Thus, indemnity plans may be able to "pick-off" lower-cost employee groups because they can better identify such groups and because they can offer lower-cost, experience-based rates to these groups. HMOs offering only community rates may not be able to attract such low-cost groups. Instead, they may increasingly attract higher-cost employers who see the average community rates of HMOs as a good deal for their higher-cost employees. Thus, a highly competitive environment could lead to a loss of profitability for many HMOs, a slower rate of growth, and a gradual trend toward a higher-risk population (Wrightson 1990). As a result of this concern, many HMOs have considered alternatives to community rating.

### Rating Changes in the 1973 HMO Act

Amendments to the HMO Act in 1981 provided for a more flexible form of community rating termed "community rating by class" (CRC). This method allows for differences in rating according to broad classes (age, sex, marital status, family size, industry, smoking status) that are known to have different utilization patterns (Sutton 1986). Members of any employer group are divided into the major classes. Rating factors based on the utilization patterns of each class are used to determine the rates for individuals in each broad class. These individual rates are then combined to form a composite rate that is equal for all members of a particular employer group. According to the law, a class could not be an employer group (i.e., one employer's employees), an occupation, or a race. CRC has demanded much more data from HMOs. However, many HMOs, particularly staff and group-model plans, have not had adequate cost data on which to determine rates by class. Often such HMOs failed to generate paperwork that could allocate physician salaries and other costs to individual enrollees. Thus, such HMOs must develop more sophisticated actuarial methods when they adopt CRC.

Employers who believed that their rates would be lower under CRC as compared to community rating have insisted on CRC. However, as more groups in lower-cost classes apply for CRC, an HMO will experience financial problems if it fails to increase the community rates to reflect the higher risk groups remaining in the community-rated pool. As some employers' rates go down because of CRC, other employers' rates go up as the community rate changes (Sutton 1986).

While CRC provided more flexibility, it did not satisfy employers' desire for experience rating from HMOs. Thus, employer groups pressed for still greater flexibility in rating requirements in the 1988 Amendments to the HMO Act. Change came in the form of "Adjusted Community Rating" (ACR). Basically, ACR is prospective experience rating where premiums are based on the historical costs of a particular group. However, the prohibitions on retrospective experience rating continued under the 1988 Amendments. Thus, the HMO's rates under ACR must reflect the projected revenue requirements of a specific employee group, and the HMO must be at risk with respect to these prospectively determined rates (Wrightson 1990).

Although HMOs may prefer the relative simplicity of community rating, they will come under increasing pressure, particularly from large employers, to provide group specific experience-based ACR. The fierce competition among HMOs and between HMO and PPOs, together with the aggressive movement of traditional insurance companies into the managed care market, will force HMOs to respond to employers' wishes.

When HMOs begin to experience rate part of their risk pool, they will be forced to examine all of it. HMOs must reflect on how prospective experience rating for one employer or client will affect the desires and the average risks of all remaining clients in the pool. It is a truism of the insurance industry that all employers believe that they have better than average experience (Traska 1989). Of course, some have to be below average with higher risk employees. Once they find that they are below average, they may wish to return to the old community rates. However, these old rates will no longer exist because the employers with the above average experience (lower risks) will have left the community pool for experience rating leaving only those with below average experience (higher risks) in the pool.

All of this indicates that HMOs will find it increasingly necessary to provide historical data for individual employer groups and to provide detailed analysis of cost and utilization patterns. This will place much greater demands on the actuarial and underwriting personnel in HMOs.

## EQUAL-EMPLOYER CONTRIBUTIONS

The 1973 HMO Act required employers to make contributions to HMOs equal in dollars to those made to indemnity or self-insured health plans offered by the employer. This requirement applied only to employers mandated under the dual-choice provisions. Those employers who voluntarily contracted with an HMO were under no equal contribution requirement. Nevertheless, employers remained opposed to the requirement.

They disliked the equal dollar requirement because they believed HMOs attracted their lower-risk, healthier employees whose health care was not as expensive as that of the higher-risk employees remaining in the indemnity plan. Thus, employers believed that they paid equal money to HMOs to provide essentially equal benefits to a group of healthier employees.

Some employers were fearful that the equal dollar contribution could undermine their intent that all employees share directly in the cost of health care. For example, employees might be expected to pay a portion of the premium for a traditional indemnity plan. However, the equal dollar contribution sometimes resulted in ''free'' HMO membership to employees even while other employees in the same company were paying a portion of the premium for the non-HMO indemnity plan. This situation could occur when the employer's portion of the traditional indemnity plan premium was so high that it exceeded the entire HMO premium (Fritz and Repko 1986).

This situation also provided an incentive for employees who were covered by their spouse's medical plan to join the ''free'' HMO even though they rarely used its services. Of course, the employer had to pay the same premium for the employees even when they failed to utilize the HMO's services.

Because of these employer concerns, the 1988 Amendments to the HMO Act modified the equal dollar contribution requirement. According to these amendments, employers must not ''financially discriminate'' against employees who join an HMO. This wording allows employers greater freedom in determining their contributions to HMO premiums. For example, employers could base their contributions to HMO and non-HMO premiums on attributes such as the age, sex and family status of the enrollees. For each enrollee in a given category, the employer would contribute an equal dollar amount regardless of the plan selected by the employee.

The amendments also allowed employers to require all employees, whether in an HMO or in non-HMO alternatives to pay part of their premiums. Specifically, if employees are required to contribute to a non-HMO plan, employees within an HMO could also be required to make a minimum contribution to the HMO premium. A contribution that does not exceed 50 percent of the contribution required for the principal non-HMO alternative is considered ''reasonable.''

Alternatively, employer contributions could be based on equal percentage contributions to HMO and non-HMO alternatives. For example, if an employer paid 80 percent of the premium for a non-HMO plan, he could also pay 80 percent of the HMO premium.

## FEDERAL QUALIFICATION PROCESS

While many employers have relied upon the qualification process as a means of encouraging quality, they are becoming increasingly dubious that the qualification process assures the delivery of quality medical services. Once an HMO has been qualified, the federal monitoring process consists solely of reviews of the financial reports of the HMO (Peres 1988). The qualification process does not produce data and documentation that quality medical care is being delivered. Thus, employers are turning increasingly to private accreditation agencies for HMOs (as described in Chapter 4) to encourage quality, and they see the federal qualification process as creating more problems than it resolves.

## DATA NEEDS

Employers are often uncomfortable with the quantity and quality of the data and reports they receive from their HMOs. As competition in the health care market increases, employers seek better data from HMOs in order to judge the effectiveness and efficiency of their services. Moreover, with adjusted community rating, employers will be searching for historical data on their employees which justifies their prospective ratings.

In the past, many HMOs simply lacked the management information systems necessary to generate data, particularly if they used community rating exclusively (Traska 1989). Staff and group-model HMOs often were unable to allocate and track costs to specific enrollees. Moreover, HMOs having data were often reluctant to share it with employers for fear that it would be misinterpreted. For example, data showing low utilization in an HMO could result from one of three possible causes: (1) the HMO is efficient and doing a good job, (2) the HMO has favorable selection, or (3) the HMO is underserving its enrollees. Two of the three are bad (Traska 1989). HMOs believe that employers often look first for the bad explanations.

In addition, many HMOs believe that employers ask for elaborate data, but when it is provided, the employers do nothing with it or fail to analyze it appropriately (InterStudy, *National Managed Care Firms* 1989).

Employers strongly supported requirements in the 1988 amendments which required federally qualified HMOs using adjusted community rating to maintain and disseminate basic data to employers.

## EMPLOYERS' EVALUATION OF HMOs

The problems and issues between employers and HMOs noted in this chapter and in previous chapters on costs and quality denote the importance of extensive employer review and evaluation of HMOs. Moreover, since employers contract with HMOs to provide health care to their employees, they have both an ethical and legal obligation to assure basic and competent service. Employees may perceive that an HMO option offered by their employer is, in effect, an endorsement of the HMO by the employer. In addition, if the marketplace approach of competition is to constrain health care costs, then the primary purchasers of such care—employers—must become more involved in the evaluation of health care delivery. Therefore, the following section concentrates on approaches and questions that employers should utilize when evaluating HMOs.

An employer's evaluation of an HMO should determine whether the HMO is both appropriate and acceptable to the employer and its employees or union (Meier and Aquilina 1982). An appropriate HMO satisfies four basic tests. First, it is accessible to the employees. Second, it provides benefits at least equal to those of plans currently provided to employees. Third, these benefits are affordable and priced appropriately. Fourth, it has a good reputation.

### Accessibility

First, the HMO must be accessible. Its service area must cover where most of the employees live and work. It must have hospitals with good reputations that are conveniently located to employees. Similarly, it must also provide 24-hour emergency service convenient for employees.

Group practice HMOs should have facilities that are within 15 to 30 minutes travel time of employees' residences or worksite. Moreover, the facilities should be accessible to public transportation. IPA model HMOs should have contracting physician offices conveniently located for most employees.

There should be sufficient physicians for the enrolled population. The ratio should not be much greater than one physician per 1,000 members unless extensive referrals are made to nonplan providers or the HMO uses physician assistants extensively (Meier and Aquilina 1982). Likewise, most of the physicians should be primary care providers and at least a majority should be accepting new patients (Ham 1989).

The employer should also ask how the primary care physicians refer patients to specialists and which specialists are available. Moreover, coordination of care is most important when a patient moves among providers.

### Benefits

After determining that an HMO has sufficient facilities and providers accessible to employees, the employer should compare the benefits provided to those employees presently receive. A chart or grid should be constructed that compares the following benefits (Varner and Christy 1986):

- Hospital care
- Physician services
- Home health care
- Routine dental services as well as dentures, crowns and bridges
- Mental health services
- Routine physicals
- Health promotion/wellness programs
- Prescription drugs
- Visual exams and eyeglasses
- Skilled or intermediate level nursing care
- Routine and nonroutine foot care
- Chiropractic care
- Hospice care

If any of the above services are not offered as basic care, are they provided as optional benefits? Are there additional optional benefits?

The employer should also compare what coverage is excluded. Are there limits on mental health and psychiatric care or for care of chronic illnesses such as diabetes or AIDS? What is the HMOs' position on experimental procedures such as organ transplants (Ham 1989)?

The employers should also compare coverage of dependents. Likewise, how do changes in the status of employees affect coverage? For example, how are disabled employees, divorced dependents, and employees eligible for medicare covered? If employees move out of the HMO's service area, how are they covered?

## Rates and Costs

The employer should ask for the HMO's community rate over the past five years. This can be compared to the rates of other HMOs in the region. Of course, the employer should ask how its group will be rated? The employer should also ask the HMO to demonstrate how it will calculate rates for its employees, employees plus spouses, and employees plus family (Ham 1989). Ask that the rates be calculated for two years. Then ask if the plan will guarantee the rates or set limits on annual increases.

The employer should ask if the HMO is willing to adapt its benefits and coverage to better meet the employer's needs and revenues. Also, the HMO's use of deductibles, copayments and coinsurance should be explored. Does it use them and for which benefits? Would it be willing to introduce them for at least some benefits?

## Reputation

If an HMO is accessible to employees and if its benefits and costs compare favorably, then its reputation should be evaluated. The employer should find out how many other employers in the region use the HMO. Check with several of the larger employers who contract with the HMO to determine their evaluations of its services and costs. Check to see if the HMO has experienced steady enrollment increases, which is one sign of employee satisfaction. Likewise, check the level of disenrollment. Also, see if the HMO has any history of malpractice suits. Determine if an employer was involved in any such suit.

Other questions that could be asked include: Is the HMO federally qualified? Does it comply with federal and state regulatory requirements? Does it have a history of noncompliance? Does the HMO have a grievance process? Are there summaries of the grievances and their dispositions? Is the HMO accredited by one of the three major accrediting bodies discussed in Chapter 4 (JCAHO, AAAHC or NCQA)?

The answers to these questions should provide a rough approximation of the reputation of the HMO and whether it is necessary to continue with a complete assessment of the HMO. If all signs are positive, a thorough evaluation of the

HMO should include a review of its management, finances, marketing, medical services, quality assurance, and utilization/cost control structures and processes (Meier and Aquilina 1982).

### Management

Employers should ask who is on the HMO's board of directors and how often it meets. Moreover, opinions could be solicited from the board members concerning evaluations of the HMO's leadership and management. Are enrollees and medical staff represented on the board? Employers should review the background and experience of key HMO personnel including the president and/or executive director, medical director, controller or finance director, and the marketing director.

Are there any parent organizations or other entities that have a direct role in policymaking and management? What is the chain of command and to whom does the medical director report?

Employers should check to see how many of the following reports are received on a monthly basis (Meier and Aquilina 1982):

1. Number of enrollees hospitalized and their expenses,
2. Participating and nonparticipating physician expenses,
3. Administrative expenses,
4. Number of members referred to nonparticipating physicians,
5. Income/Expense statement,
6. Comparison of actual costs vs. budget revenues,
7. For an IPA, utilization rates of health services for each individual physician.

The existence of these reports is a good indication of the HMOs intent to develop an effective management information system.

### Finance

Given the recent failures of HMOs, employers need to obtain as much financial information as possible about an HMO. Is it for-profit or nonprofit? The nonprofits' failure rate has tended to be lower than profits. Likewise, the nonprofits tend to be the older, more established, larger plans. Also, IPAs have been experiencing the greatest financial problems in recent years while staff models tended to have the best liquidity.

Employers should know who will be at risk for losses incurred by an HMO. If the HMO is part of a larger national or regional corporation, does a certain percentage of the HMO's profits go to the parent organization? Does the HMO have to pay the parent company for administrative services? If the national firm goes bankrupt, what are the obligations of the HMO to the parent company (Ham 1989)?

The employer should ask what portion of the HMO's operating risk is reinsured. HMOs, particularly smaller ones, often have stop-loss reinsurance for protection against large unanticipated claims. If the HMOs have reinsurance, they have been scrutinized and accepted by insurers. If they do not have reinsurance, it could be because they did not apply for it, or could not get it. In either case, the implications are not good.

If the HMO fails, there should be assurances that the enrollees and the employer will not be held responsible by providers for the debts incurred by the HMO.

The employer should obtain the HMO's financial statements for the past several years. Review of these statements should give an employer an approximate sense of the overall financial condition of the HMO. Has the HMO been making or losing money? Have the profits or losses been increasing or decreasing over the past three to five years? What have been the trends in net worth? Are current assets greater than current liabilities? What are the long-term debts and liabilities of the HMO and at what rate are these to be repaid?

What are the HMO's current operating expenses? What percentage of these are covered by capitation, fee-for-service income, draws on credit, or other income? Is the HMO currently breaking even? If not, when will it? What enrollment and premium level are needed to break even? Are these realistic given current levels (Meier and Aquilina 1982)? What are the ratios of medical institutional expenses and physician expenses to premium revenues? Have the rates been increasing, decreasing or remaining constant? What are the ratios of administrative expenses to premium revenues? Have these been increasing or decreasing? These ratios should probably be in the range of 35 to 60 percent for institutional care, 40 to 60 percent for physician services, and 8 to 20 percent for administrative expenses (Ham 1989; Meier and Aquilina 1982).

The employer should also review the history of rate increases in the HMO over the past several years. Of course, these should be lower than the average indemnity plan rate increases in the area.

Finally, the employer should inquire about the HMO's projections of future enrollment and rate levels. What rate of hospital utilization supports the premium projections? If the HMO does not have these projections, it may not be planning very well. Ask what contingency plans it may have if enrollment is only 75 percent of projection or if hospital utilization is significantly higher than projections (Meier and Aquilina 1982)?

### Marketing and Enrollment

As noted in Chapter 3, HMOs can use marketing strategies to encourage favorable selection of the healthier low-risk employees into the HMOs. To prevent this possibility, employers should carefully review and oversee how the

HMO intends to market its services to employees. Essentially, the employer should ensure that all employees receive the same information about the basic and supplemental benefits of the HMO, and the HMO's procedures for selecting a physician, obtaining referrals, and arranging routine and emergency care. The employer should probably coordinate workplace orientation sessions for all employees in which the new plan is discussed by both HMO and employer representatives. If the employer wants as many employees to enroll in the HMO as possible (which will be the most cost-efficient), then the employer should make it convenient for employees to attend orientation sessions.

The employer should review all brochures and written material to be presented by the HMO to assure clarity and to ensure equal appeal to employees across all demographic groups. Employees should be provided with the names and phone numbers of individuals to contact for more information about the plan.

### Medical Services

The employer should determine which of the following services are provided directly by the HMO or through outside contracts or through referrals to noncontractors: hospital nursing facilities, primary physician care, specialists (by type), prescriptions, laboratory tests, X rays, ambulance services, mental health, vision and dental care, and chemical dependency. It is preferable that as many services as possible come directly from the HMO. This is particularly true for primary care physicians.

Moreover, the employer should ask how physicians are paid? Salary? Capitation? Fee-for-service? Are bonuses given to primary physicians for lower utilization? Are the bonus pools based on individual or group performance? How are physicians penalized for utilization of medical services? Are all physicians required to carry malpractice insurance? Answers to these questions can help one to assess the physicians' incentive to control costs and/or promote quality (Ham 1989). The physicians should be at some risk in order to control utilization. Likewise, the employer should inquire about the HMO's method of payment to hospitals. Are full charges paid? Discounted charges? Per diem? Capitation? The method of payment will affect the hospitals' incentives to control utilization and costs. Again, it is better that the hospital be at some risk in order to reduce utilization.

The employer should be particularly concerned about how the HMO will coordinate provision of primary care services to patients. How will the HMO assist the enrollee in selecting a physician? Can enrollees see the credentials of physicians? Will the primary physician coordinate all of the enrollee's medical care in the HMO?

A number of other questions concerning the quality of providers should be asked. These are discussed in Chapter 4.

## Quality Assurance

As efforts to control the costs of medical care accelerate, pressure to compromise the quality of medical services also increases. Thus, it is important that an employer insist on quality as well as efficiency from an HMO. A thorough discussion of quality in HMOs as well as what employers can do to promote quality health care delivery are discussed in Chapter 4. Areas of concern discussed in Chapter 4 include an HMO's quality assurance plan, quality contracts with providers (physicians and hospitals), required provider credentials and quality criteria for selecting physicians, renewal of provider contracts, and quality reviews of providers such as physical therapists, chiropractors, pharmacies, and nursing agencies. Questions concerning all of these areas should be addressed to the HMO.

The employer should also obtain copies of any enrollee satisfaction studies done by the HMO, as well as annual disenrollment rates, and physician turnover rates. If these rates are high, explanations should be sought. The employer should also ask for summaries of grievances over the past several years as well as the HMO's response to these grievances. Likewise, information concerning malpractice suits against the HMO's providers should be solicited.

The employer should determine if the HMO is accredited by one of the organizations noted in Chapter 4. If the HMO is not accredited, why? Is it seeking accreditation? If not, why?

## Utilization Review

For both quality and costs purposes, employers should ensure that the HMO practices good utilization review. It should conduct preadmission certification of nonemergency hospital admissions. Here the HMO reviews the facts of a case to determine if hospitalization is appropriate. Likewise, it should require concurrent review where the appropriateness and medical necessity of hospital admissions and stays are reviewed while the episode of illness is in progress. The HMO should also practice retrospective review which occurs after the patient is discharged from the hospital. Again, it determines whether hospitalization and treatment were appropriate. Precertification of referrals by primary physicians to specialists can also be a useful utilization control providing the HMO has reliable criteria for determining what referrals are appropriate. The employer should ask the HMO to detail how it conducts all of these reviews and certifications.

The employer should also obtain the non-Medicare statistics on inpatient days per 1,000 enrollees, hospital admissions per 1,000 enrollees, and average length of stay. These statistics should be compared with other local utilization statistics from groups whose demographics are roughly similar to those of the employer's employees (Ham 1989).

The HMO should routinely review the practice patterns of physicians. Here the HMO tracks physicians' treatments of illnesses to see if some doctors "over utilize" or "under utilize" compared to other physicians in the plan. Feedback from these reviews should be given to physicians. Contracts for physicians with practice patterns consistently outside the norms should be reviewed closely. Employers should ask the HMO how it utilizes data on practice patterns to change physicians' behavior.

Employers should ask the HMO if it reviews the utilization patterns of physicians during a probation/evaluation period in the HMO. Are physicians ever removed for deviant utilization patterns?

If utilization controls are to work, the HMO should place the physician at some risk for use of medical services. A recent survey of HMOs revealed that over 75 percent placed the individual physician at risk for primary services and 50 percent put the individual physician at risk for specialist treatment (InterStudy, *National Managed Care Firms* 1989). Employers should ask the HMO to explain how physicians are placed at risk in the HMO.

In recent years, costs for mental health and chemical dependency care, emergency services, and pharmacy services have been increasing dramatically. Employers should make inquiries into the HMO's specific methods of controlling utilization in these areas.

## CONCLUSION

In recent years, we have seen dramatic increases in health care costs that are likely to continue as a result of new technologies (heart/lung transplants, CAT scans), new diseases (AIDS), and government mandated employer-financed benefits (treatment for mental illness and chemical dependency).

Likewise, more employers are becoming concerned about the eventual impact of the new method of accounting for future retiree medical liabilities as proposed by the Financial Accounting Standard Board (FASB). The FASB proposal requires companies to record retiree medical benefits on an accrual basis as a form of deferred compensation that must be expensed while employees are producing revenues. For larger companies, this change could produce an annual profit drop as large as 15 percent. As a result of these pressures, employers will increasingly turn to managed care providers, such as HMOs, to control costs.

Many employers' concerns about HMOs should subside as a result of the 1988 amendments to the HMO Act of 1973. These amendments provide the needed flexibility for HMOs to respond to employers' wishes. Thus, at employers urging, many HMOs will increasingly move from community rating to some form of experience rating.

Employers with many employees will seek ever more information from HMOs concerning utilization, quality, and costs. They will demand documented results for their health care dollar. The larger HMOs will probably be best able to respond to these employer requests. Therefore, large HMOs will continue to have a competitive advantage over smaller ones. Likewise, HMOs and PPOs will engage in vigorous competition which the HMOs will probably win because they are structurally better able to control costs. Indeed, many non-HMO managed care plans will probably begin to look more and more like HMOs even though they will not call themselves HMOs.

Employers will dramatically reduce the number of health care options provided to employees. Reducing the number of options will make it easier for employers to manage data and track utilization and expenditures. It will also ease the "skimming problem" and facilitate administration of laws such as Section 89 of the 1986 Tax Reform Act, which prohibits discrimination in benefits offered to high and low-income employees. Of course, it is less difficult to document nondiscrimination when there are only one or two plans offered to employees.

More employers may "sole source" all of their health care with an open-ended HMO that provides enrollees a choice at point of service between the HMO's providers and an indemnity plan that is often affiliated with the HMO. Such an arrangement can overcome the employees' initial reluctance to accept an HMO. Of course, the HMO and the employer hope the employees save money by using the HMO providers.

If health care costs continue to rise at dramatic rates, employers will make it increasingly less attractive for their employees to receive care outside the HMO by increasing the deductibles and copayments for such care. Also, as employees become more comfortable with HMOs, employers concerned over health care costs may urge HMOs to apply copayments to more HMO benefits and to adopt deductibles. Such payments will contribute directly to reduction of costs and, just as importantly, discourage utilization.

In the health care arena of providers, patients, employers, and managed care organizations, the employers have potentially the most influence. They pay the bills. Perhaps employers will not long continue to pay double digit increases in health care costs without first adopting more dramatic steps to control the costs and/or shift them to their employees.

Employers must try to show employees that if the cost of health care continues to escalate, the employees will have to pay for it with lower salaries, fewer jobs, or both. Moreover, employers cannot hope to control costs unless they limit the choice of providers. Eventually, employees facing large deductibles and copayments when using outside providers may arrive at the same conclusion. Then both employer and employees may push to place providers more at risk when medical care costs exceed revenues.

HMOs with select panels of providers, internal case management procedures, utilization controls, and efficient data management systems can be very useful weapons in the employers' fight against cost increases. Over the longer term, HMOs with these attributes will be valued by employers.

# 6

# HMOs and Providers

The success of any HMO is critically dependent on its relations with providers, particularly physicians. An HMO's doctors are primarily responsible for its reputation in the community and its ability to recruit new members. Moreover, since physicians control 60 to 70 percent of all health care expenditures, their cooperation is absolutely essential in an HMO's efforts to control utilization and costs.

The wide variety in medical practice patterns (described below) permit considerable opportunity for HMOs to influence how doctors practice medicine. HMOs use numerous methods to influence doctors' practice patterns. These methods include selective recruitment, education, feedback, various payment modes, and administrative guidelines.

## PHYSICIANS' PRACTICE PATTERNS

If medicine were an exact science and if all physicians' practice patterns were very similar, then HMOs would have little opportunity to influence their physicians' practice of medicine. However, there is ample evidence of wide variation in medical practice. For example, there are huge variations in surgical rates for hysterectomies, tonsillectomies, proctalectomies, and other surgeries even within small geographical areas (Wennberg and Gittelsohn 1982). Nonsurgical rates vary even more than surgical rates. For example, hospitalization rates differ dramatically for various diagnostic categories including gastroenteritis (18-fold differences), lower respiratory tract infections (15-fold differences) and upper respiratory tract infections (8-fold differences) (Connell et al. 1981).

After patients are hospitalized or have surgery, they receive widely varying ancillary services for the same diagnoses. Moreover, there is variation in the use of laboratory tests even when there are controls for case mix (Roos 1982; Greenwald et al. 1984). Likewise, prescription of drugs varies by region and physician (Hartzema and Christenson 1983). Similarly, rates of referral to consultants also vary (Rothert et al. 1984).

Many studies have revealed dramatic differences among nations in the number of hospital admissions and surgical rates per capita, length of stay in the hospital, and use of ancillary services (Abel-Smith 1984; Epstein et al. 1984).

While many of these studies attempted to control for case-mix differences in the treatment of different patients by different doctors, it is difficult to perfectly control for severity of disease and other confounding variables. Nevertheless, the collective weight of such studies on medical practice variation suggests that while some variation is caused by case-mix differences, much results from differences in physicians' practice patterns (Eisenberg 1986).

This variation suggests that much medical care may be unnecessary. Indeed there is considerable evidence of unnecessary utilization in ordering diagnostic tests, laboratory tests, prescriptions, hospital days, surgery, and nursing care (Eisenberg 1986).

Unnecessary medical care causes concern because most of the medical care is paid by third-party payers (e.g., insurers, employers, and government). Thus, unnecessary health care received by one person is paid for by many others who share the pooled risk. Since medical care is viewed as a need, not a luxury, its use should be dependent on real need and not result from the peculiar proclivities of individual doctors, or the patient's preferences unless the individual doctor or patient is willing to pay for the unneeded, but desired care (Eisenberg 1986). Moreover, unnecessary medical care can be dangerous as well as wasteful.

Medical practice patterns result from the interplay of a number of complex factors as perceived by the physician including (1) the perceived probability of disease, (2) the potential clinical benefits and costs, (3) the economic costs to the patient, (4) the economic benefits to the physician and his organization, (5) the potential benefit or cost to the physician in his satisfaction with his practice, (6) the potential impact on the physicians' self-image or status in the community, and (7) the potential benefits and costs to society (Eisenberg 1986).

Doctors evaluate all of these factors consciously or unconsciously when deciding whether to prescribe medical care, and it is within this complex set of factors that HMOs' attempt to model or change the behavior of their physicians.

## HMOs' ATTEMPT TO INFLUENCE PHYSICIANS' BEHAVIOR

HMOs can influence their physicians' behavior in a number of ways. Of course, HMOs, particularly group and staff-model HMOs, try to recruit doctors who will be comfortable with the style of medicine practiced in HMOs. Thus, HMOs first method of guiding physician behavior is to select the right kind of doctor.

Another primary way in which HMOs attempt to guide behavior is through education and feedback to doctors. This may involve information about the HMO's goals and objectives as well as the competitive environment faced by the HMO. It may also entail feedback about each physician's utilization pattern compared to other physicians' patterns.

A third major method that HMOs use to affect physician behavior is the choice and operation of financial incentive plans. Some HMOs may use capitation, while others use salaries or modified fee-for-service with risk pools.

Other methods to control behavior include use of physicians as leaders and role models, physician participation in peer oversight committees, and numerous administrative controls designed to control utilization and quality. These methods are discussed in greater detail below.

### HMOs' Recruitment of Physicians

Perhaps the best way for HMOs to promote the practice patterns they desire is to exercise great care in admitting physicians into HMOs. The increase in the supply of physicians in recent years has made it considerably easier for HMOs to attract physicians, and most can afford to be more selective. Many staff/group-model HMOs may admit only 60 to 80 percent of those physicians who apply (Fox and Heinen 1987).

Of course, this is less true in areas where the number of physicians per capita remains significantly below the national average. As one might expect, physicians are more likely to join an HMO in areas where HMOs market penetration is highest. Therefore, physicians in highly populated urban areas are three times as likely to join an HMO as are rural doctors (Rosenbach et al. 1988). Likewise, the number of physicians per capita tend to be higher in wealthier urban areas. Thus, the greater level of competition among doctors in the more highly populated, more affluent areas, where many physicians are located and where large employers are likely to sponsor HMOs, encourages higher levels of physician participation in HMOs.

Recent research indicates that approximately one-third of all physicians participate in an HMO. Approximately 18 percent are in group or staff-model HMOs and another 14 or 15 percent in IPAs (Rosenbach et al. 1988). IPAs have attracted the greater number of doctors in recent years. This rapid increase reflects IPAs' more relaxed approach to physician recruitment and admission. Some IPAs, particularly those that are physician-sponsored, may admit any doctor in good standing of the local medical society and with privileges at a participating hospital. Admission may be on a first-come, first-served basis (Fox and Heinen 1987).

It is unfortunate that IPAs often have the most informal approach to recruitment of physicians. Since IPAs are the most decentralized of all HMOS and lack the formal rules and hierarchy often found in staff/group models, they are most in need of physicians who share a common philosophy and commitment to the

HMO approach to medicine. Yet there is often no concerted effort to attract such physicians into IPAs.

Generally, HMOs place greatest efforts in attracting primary care physicians, particularly family practitioners, internists, and pediatricians. These primary care physicians often serve as the essential "gatekeepers" in the HMO. They are responsible for referring patients to specialists and must agree to most hospital admissions. Thus, they are essential in HMOs' attempts to control utilization and quality. These specialists plus obstetricians/gynecologists account for nearly half of all HMO physicians. Interestingly, however, general practitioners tend not to participate in HMOs. Only 18 percent of all GPs are in HMOs, and most of these are in less structured IPAs.

One reason for the lower number of GPs in HMOs is that most tend to be older and/or in solo practice. Younger physicians are much more likely to join an HMO. Almost 40 percent of all physicians under age 35 participate in HMOs. This participation rate declines steadily with age. As the supply of physicians has increased, younger physicians, who are just beginning their careers, have increasingly looked to HMOs as one method of establishing a practice and building regular income (Goodman and Swartwout 1984).

Older physicians, with well established practices, may not feel the competitive pressure as much as younger physicians (Rosenbach et al. 1988). Also, older physicians may be looking to decrease rather than increase their practices.

Another reason why younger physicians participate in HMOs is that HMOs often recruit younger physicians more aggressively. HMOs assume that physicians with less established practice patterns are less rigid and more amenable to an HMO's influence. Conversely, many older physicians with solo practices are more philosophically opposed to HMOs and are more concerned about maintaining their independence. Indeed, the main reason which doctors give for not joining an HMO is that they wish to maintain their independence. Older physicians are much more inclined to give this reason (Rosenbach et al. 1988).

HMOs, particularly staff and group-model HMOs, often recruit female doctors. Staff or group-model HMOs hire many pediatricians who have a higher percentage of females than do the other specialties. Women tend to like the more regular work hours and greater free time provided by prepaid group practice. The desire for shorter, more predictable work hours is the chief reason given by female physicians for joining an HMO (Rosenbach et al. 1988). This is consistent with research which indicates that female doctors work fewer hours than do male physicians (Mitchell 1984). Apparently, female doctors value free time and regular work hours over the additional income from seeing more patients.

HMOs that carefully select physicians solicit much information from physicians seeking entry into an HMO. The application form often requests information about state licensure, specialist training, and board certification. It may also ask about hospital privileges at participating hospitals, office hours, how calls after office hours are processed, and how referrals to specialists are made.

If information on the application seems appropriate, a site visit and interview will be arranged. The site visit reviews the location of the office vis-a-vis the HMO's enrollees. Some HMOs may accept a physician because the office location can be used in marketing the HMO to an employer and its employees.

The site visit is also used to check the attractiveness and cleanliness of the facilities. Moreover, the physician's recordkeeping and quality assurance systems will be reviewed. In addition, there may be a sample review of the charts to assess standards of care in the HMO.

Interviews are primarily used to discern the attitudes of physicians toward HMOs. Of course, HMOs do not wish to employ physicians who are hostile toward HMOs but who feel they must join because of competitive pressure. Likewise, most HMOs do not want the "entrepreneur" type of doctor who is seeking to build a large income out of his or her practice (Meier and Tillotson 1978). Moreover, the HMO, particularly the group and staff-model HMOs, do not want a doctor whose ego is too large to accept continuous oversight and review by peers and by utilization and quality review personnel.

### Education and Feedback to Physicians in HMOs

HMOs have numerous ways to educate and provide feedback to physicians to control utilization. Although education and feedback are conceptually very similar, the two are not identical. As used here, education is giving new information to physicians in the hope that it will modify their behavior. Feedback is informing physicians about *their individual behavior* as it compares to others.

Education by HMOs often entails information concerning how less expensive care (drugs, tests, and so on) can be used without affecting quality of care. Most doctors are not well-informed about the costs of care (Robertson 1980). Research shows that approximately two-thirds of physicians do not know the costs of tests that they order (Thomas and Davis 1987). If they knew the costs, they might be less likely to order tests in cases where the need for them is not compelling. Programs to educate doctors about costs report decreases in utilization of approximately 30 percent, particularly in the use of diagnostic tests (Eisenberg 1986).

The effectiveness of such programs sharply declines over time if there are not consistent, continuous reminders. For example, computer reminders of the costs of tests each time they were ordered have reduced the number of tests ordered. However, once the reminders were eliminated, the number of tests ordered returned to higher levels (Tierney et al. 1990). Thus, education, to be effective, must be continuously reinforced and be part of a long-term, permanent education effort.

HMOs often use feedback of a physician's individual behavior in comparison with the behavior of other physicians to influence his or her practice style. HMOs may inform individual physicians of many comparisons including their:

a. enrollee load compared to the average in the HMO,
b. number of office visits per a given time period compared to the HMO average,

c. average amount of money received per visit compared to the HMO average,
d. number of specialty referrals as a percent of total visits compared to the HMO average,
e. number of specific tests ordered expressed as a ratio of the number of visits compared to the HMO average,
f. number and types of prescriptions as compared to the HMO average,
g. number of admissions to the hospital and days of care for a given time period compared to the HMO average.

These kinds of feedback combined with educational efforts designed to control utilization notify "outliers" that they are outside the norms, and provides information about how to reduce utilization.

Research indicates that education and feedback are most useful in HMOs when they come from other physicians (Eisenberg 1986). Thus, the roles of the HMO's medical director and other physician leaders are critical in an HMO's educational efforts. Formal and informal, personal, face-to-face consultation among respected colleagues is perhaps the most effective educational method to change physician behavior (Stross et al. 1983).

Formal and informal peer pressure combined with financial incentives have produced change in practice styles of HMO physicians. This can be seen in lower rates of surgery and hospitalization as well as different attitudes concerning tests and prescriptions (Eisenberg 1986). This collegial oversight, consultation, and pressure are more likely to take place within the social structure of a staff or group-model HMO. In these HMOs, physicians are often more proximate to one another and more likely to interact on a continuing basis. Conversely, IPAs which are composed of many solo practice physicians who have administrative arrangements with an IPA but little direct contact with other physicians in the IPA, will have significantly less opportunity to profit from their peers' advice.

In summary, Eisenberg (1986) concludes that education and feedback are most likely to be successful in changing physicians' behavior when they are individualized, when doctors are compared with their peers, and when the information is delivered personally by a doctor in a position of clinical leadership. Moreover, feedback/education is most successful when it concerns a problem about which doctors have reached consensus concerning the appropriate standards of practice.

## Financial Incentives in HMOs and Physician Behavior

There is ample evidence that doctors' desire for income can affect their practice styles. When fee controls were established under the Economic Stabilization Program in 1971, doctors increased their income by increasing the quantity of their services, by shifting to a higher-priced mix of services, and by "unbundling services" (i.e., charging separately for items previously combined under one charge) (Holahan et al. 1979; Yett et al. 1983).

Likewise, reduction of medicare payment schedules in Colorado resulted in the provision of more intensive services (Rice 1983). Similarly, the Rand Health Care Experiment showed that when allowable charges for office visits were reduced, physicians substituted laboratory tests for time spent with patients (Danzon 1984).

Three-fourths of all physicians who join an HMO say they did so to increase their patient load and to have more regular income (Rosenbach et al. 1988). Thus, if doctors join an HMO for income, and if their desire for income can affect their practice styles, it is reasonable to expect HMOs to manipulate the methods of reimbursing their physicians in the hope of influencing how they practice medicine. HMOs use a variety of physician payment methods including:

a. Capitation—the physician receives a set fee per enrollee for a given period of time;
b. Salary—the physician receives a regular salary at a constant rate;
c. Fee-For-Service—the physician receives a set fee from a schedule of fees for specific services;
d. Withhold—a percentage of the physician payment is retained until the end of the accounting period to cover any deficit incurred for delivered health services;
e. Bonus—the physician shares a portion of any surplus remaining in the withhold fund after any deficits are covered.

Capitation is the most common method of payment in HMOs with approximately half of all HMOs using it (*InterStudy Edge* 1989; Hillman et al. 1989). A modified fee-for-service with a percentage of the fees placed in a withhold account is used by approximately one-third of all HMOs. Salaries are used by about 10 percent of all HMOs and a combination of methods are used by the rest.

The dominant type of payment system differs among the various types of HMOs. Network models use capitation overwhelmingly (77 percent); IPAs and group HMOs are split between capitation and fee-for-service; and staff-model HMOs rely almost exclusively (79 percent) on salary-based payment (Hillman et al. 1989).

*Salaried Physicians in HMOs*. Most staff-model plans pay physicians a straight salary. Thus, the physicians do not have any direct fee-for-service incentives to provide more medical care than is necessary. In addition, there are other methods for controlling utilization in such HMOs. Budgets are carefully reviewed and utilization statistics are compared in order to control both utilization and productivity.

Physicians are more carefully selected in staff-model HMOs in order to assure proper ''fit'' between the physicians' attitudes and goals and those of the HMO (Fox and Heinen 1987). Moreover, staff-model HMOs are more likely to have an environment in which interaction with peers and on-site specialists promote greater informal discussion of cases and fewer referrals (Fox and Heinen 1987).

Since a salary system may not be a strong incentive for greater productivity, other methods of promoting productivity have been employed in such systems. For example, the normal or expected appointment schedule or the expected number of patients a doctor should see per week are used to control the productivity of salaried physicians.

Some HMOs with salary systems have experimented with bonuses in which physicians are paid a percentage, say 85 percent, of their normal salary for their specialty and seniority with additional compensation accruing according to the number of enrollees for whom they are responsible (Fox and Heinen 1987). Other HMOs may offer year-end bonuses to salaried physicians if costs were kept below projections. The impact of such bonuses on physicians' behavior probably depends on the size of the bonus pool, how many doctors share in it, and the size of the individual bonus as a percentage of the doctor's salary. The fewer doctors who participate in the pool and the larger the bonus as a percentage of salary, the greater its probable impact.

Bonuses remain a relatively small portion (less than 5 percent) of the income of physicians who are employed by staff or group-model HMOs (Rosenbach et al. 1988). Thus, it should not be too surprising that recent research indicates the distribution of bonuses had little effect on productivity or utilization (Hillman et al. 1989).

*Fee-For-Service Systems in HMOs*. Fee-for-service payments are used by some IPA model HMOs. In an attempt to control utilization, most IPAs (82 percent) withhold a portion (usually 11 to 20 percent) of the fees (Hillman 1989). This withhold is used to cover deficits that the HMO may incur when total health care costs are greater than premium revenues. The withhold may be used to cover referrals to specialists or to cover portions of hospitalization costs.

The effectiveness of such withholds in controlling utilization depends on several factors. First, if the withhold is computed on a collective or group basis, then each individual physician may recognize only a tenuous relationship between his or her individual actions and the financial state of the collective withhold pool. Indeed, the individual physician may conclude that his individual interest is maximized by generating more services and fees rather than worrying about how his overutilization could deplete the collective risk pool.

The withhold will not be very effective if the individual physician has few HMO patients among his total patient load. Approximately 13 percent of all physicians who participate in HMOs have no HMO patients. In other words, these doctors join HMOs but receive no patients or income from them (Rosenbach et al. 1988). Obviously, these physicians will be little influenced by HMOs' incentive plans.

Among the doctors who receive any income from HMOs, the average percent of their net income received from the HMO is about 30 percent (Rosenbach et al. 1988). The higher this percentage, the more likely the withhold will be effective in reducing utilization. But if we assume that the withhold is often no higher than 20 percent, then only approximately 6 percent or less (20 × 30 percent) of a physician's net income would be affected by the withhold.

When one realizes that many physicians' collection rates for regular, non-HMO fee-for-service patients is little better than 90 percent, the 6 percent of net income at risk through the HMO may not appear to be much of a disincentive to utilization (Meier and Tillotson 1978). This is particularly true if the risk pool is spread across a large number of doctors. Given these limitations in the use of withholds, perhaps it is not too surprising that recent research indicates that they have little impact on utilization (Hillman et al. 1989).

*Capitation in HMOs.* Capitation is the dominant method that HMOs use to pay physicians. It is used overwhelmingly in network model HMOs and in almost half of all IPAs and group model HMOs. With capitation, the physicians receive a payment for each enrollee. Two-thirds of the HMOs that use capitation also withhold a portion of the payments to cover referral and hospitalization costs.

When the health care costs exceed the capitated payments, the physicians "eat" the loss and incur the risk. However, when the costs are less than the payments, the physicians enjoy the surplus.

Capitation payments can be made to individual physicians or to groups of physicians who in turn may pay salaries or fee-for-services to physicians in the group. When payments are made to each physician, the physician assumes all of the risk. When capitation payments are made to the group, the risk is pooled across numerous physicians.

Apparently, the number of physicians being placed at individual risk is increasing. In a 1986 survey, only 18 percent of the HMOs made capitation payments to individual physicians (Gold 1988). However, a 1989 survey showed that almost 60 percent of responding HMOs paid capitation payments to their individual physicians. Another 22 percent made capitation payments to physician groups which then reimbursed individual physicians on a nonrisk basis (*InterStudy Edge* 1989). Just over 11 percent made capitation payments to both the group and the individual.

Critics have been concerned about placing individual physicians at risk (Welch 1987). They believe that the pressure on individual physicians to underutilize health care would be too great if they assumed most of the risk. When risks are shared by a medical group, with many patients, it is difficult for individual physicians to see how the treatment of any one patient could affect the collective risk pool. Therefore, physicians' decisions concerning any single patient's care is more likely to be governed by medical need rather than economic concerns. However, if the risk pool is no larger than one physician's patients, the nexus between the treatment offered to any single patient and the financial state of the risk pool could become very pronounced in the physician's mind. Thus, critics argue that the physician may be tempted to compromise medical care for economic gain.

There are several methods to reduce physicians' risks. Capitation rates can be fixed according to the age and sex of enrollees. In this way, the capitation payments would more nearly parallel the probable expenditures for the enrollees. Second, over half of HMOs provide stop-loss insurance which insures a physician or group against expenditures above a predetermined amount for any one patient (*InterStudy Edge* 1989). Third, enrollees with very expensive diseases (e.g., AIDS, renal disease) could be financed in a different way.

Despite these protections against physician risks, there are continuing concerns that capitation, particularly where the individual physician has his or her own risk pool, will result in underutilization. Thus, HMOs that use capitation employ numerous means to assure sufficient utilization including quality assurance/utilization review (82 percent), grievance procedures (25 percent), patient satisfaction surveys (19 percent), and physician selection processes (11 percent) (*InterStudy Edge* 1989).

HMOs use a variety of methods to establish capitation rates. The most common methods base rates on demographic characteristics (age, sex) and on the geographic location of the plan's enrollees (*InterStudy Edge* 1989). The next most frequently cited method is the past experience of the physician group and the HMO's experience.

### HMOs and Primary Care Physicians as Gatekeepers

HMOs have been interested in using primary-care physicians to become coordinators and financial managers of medical care for their patients (Moore et al. 1983). Under this arrangement, the primary care physician receives a capitated amount per enrollee per month. A withhold of varying amounts is used to cover referrals to specialists and perhaps hospitalization. If there is a surplus in the withhold, the physician would receive a portion or all of it. In theory, this approach has certain merits. It supports the primary physician's role in maintaining continuity of patient care, a long-standing problem in HMOs. It could also provide utilization control.

However, there have been some problems with the gatekeeper concept. First, because the withhold is relatively small, say 10–15 percent of the capitation payment, the incentive is too small for the primary physician to be concerned about referrals and hospitalization. Second, the primary physicians often had only a few HMO patients among their total patient load. Thus, again, the physicians did not have sufficient stake in the HMO's operation, whether measured by the percentage of the withhold or the number of patients, to justify much concern about referrals and hospitalization (Moore et al. 1983).

If the withhold is computed on an individual physician basis, the primary physician is subject to random expensive cases that cannot be spread over a larger group of physicians and a bigger patient population. Thus, primary physicians could be practicing conservative medicine as they were intended to do only to realize that the existence or lack of one or two expensive cases determined the deficit or surplus in their withhold account at the end of the year (Moore et al. 1983).

On the other hand, when the primary care physicians' withholds are pooled across a large number of physicians, then everyone's responsibility becomes no one's responsibility. Moreover, if there is no organizational management, such as a group practice, to provide practice style norms and guidelines, the group pool can be depleted by widely varying practice styles (Moore et al. 1983).

Primary care physicians generally have inadequate time to monitor and control hospitalization and the performance of procedures by specialists. Also, they face an obvious conflict of interest in such situations, particularly if the HMO has not exercised considerable care to select specialists whose practice styles reflect the HMO's philosophy.

The gatekeeper approach will probably work best when used within a medical group structure where there are established practice norms and informal and formal mechanisms to control both utilization and quality. Moreover, the primary-care physicians should have a high percentage of their patient load in the HMO. In addition, the HMO should use great care in selecting both the primary-care physicians and the specialists, and should assure that both understand their roles and how they should interrelate.

The use of individual physician risk pools places too heavy a financial risk on the individual primary physician. There probably should be collective pools based on sizable withholds of 20–50 percent (Ramsdell 1985). Further, utilization review guidelines should reinforce appropriate practice styles to assure a more uniform approach among all gatekeepers and to assure that quality is not sacrificed for financial gain.

Finally, primary-care gatekeepers will need considerable administrative assistance to assure adequate monitoring of hospitalization and referrals. If they have a sizable patient load, it is doubtful that they can perform this function in addition to the delivery of primary care.

## Administrative Controls and Physicians' Behavior

HMOs use a variety of rules and guidelines to guide their physicians' practice of medicine. Many of the rules involve prior certification or authorization for medical care. Most all elective surgery in HMOs must have prior authorization. Likewise, admission into hospitals for elective surgery at night or over the weekend is not usually permitted. Mandatory second opinions are requested for many surgeries. Also, there are lists of surgeries and other procedures that must be performed on an outpatient basis.

Prior authorization is often necessary for ambulatory services such as CAT scans, home health care, drugs, speech therapy, and mental health counseling. Similarly, referrals to specialists often require prior approval.

Concurrent review of inpatient care occurs simultaneously with inpatient care. Utilization review nurses monitor admissions and certify lengths-of-stay based on diagnostic-specific criteria and standards. They continue chart reviews of patients and discuss the patients' status with hospital staff to determine the earliest discharge date.

Retrospective review of some cases which for one reason or another fall outside predetermined norms occurs in many HMOs. Such reviews may reveal if some physicians have a pattern of overuse.

Apparently these guidelines and reviews do have an impact on physician behavior. Recent research indicates such practices reduced inpatient admissions by 12 percent, inpatient days by 8 percent, hospital expenditures by 12 percent, and total medical expenditures by over 8 percent (Feldstein 1988).

### Summary of HMOs' Attempt to Influence Physician Behavior

It is difficult to say which of the various methods used by HMOs to influence physician behavior is most effective. Most studies of changes in the doctors' practice patterns have not had good controls. For example, financial incentives may have been changing simultaneously with educational and feedback efforts. Likewise, case-mix differences and differences in severity of illness may have confounded results.

Differences in practice styles that are attributed to interventions could be due to regression to the mean where outliers simply move closer to the norm of a group. If the intent of the change efforts were to persuade outliers to be more like the group, the effort could be judged a success. However, it could also be a statistical artifact of regression to the mean. Further, if an intervention was intended to change the practice patterns of all physicians but only changed the behavior of outliers, its success would be unclear.

There have been few prospective, longitudinal studies of changes in physicians' practice styles. Hence, it is difficult to know if observed changes were statistical accidents or if they were lasting changes. Finally, few studies reveal cost-benefit data on attempts to change doctors' behavior. Is the economic gain from changes in physicians' behavior greater than the costs of the program to induce such change?

HMOs will be most successful in influencing physician behavior when multiple methods to affect change are utilized and when these methods reinforce one another. Thus, financial incentives and education are most effective when the most receptive physicians have been recruited into an HMO. Similarly, feedback is most effective when reinforced by financial incentives and administrative reviews. Therefore, an HMO will be most successful in influencing its physicians' practice styles when it knows what style it seeks and when it integrates recruitment, compensation, education and administrative reviews to promote that style.

## HMOs AND HOSPITALS

Hospitals and HMOs often pursue conflicting goals. HMOs try not to hospitalize their members while hospitals seek patients. The contour and context of this naturally antagonistic relationship are often shaped by the nature of the local hospital market. The ways in which the market influences relations between HMOs and hospitals are discussed in this section. Also, the types of contracts between hospitals and HMOs are discussed as well as those factors that limit an HMO's influence over hospitals.

## The Local Hospital Market

The relationship between an HMO and a hospital is shaped by the hospital's local market characteristics and the level and type of competition within that market. A hospital without much competition from another hospital is less likely to respond favorably to an HMO's request for risk-sharing or discounts. Similarly, a hospital with low capacity and high occupancy will not make many concessions to an HMO. On the other hand, a hospital with high capacity, low occupancy and viable competitors is an excellent candidate for an HMO contract (Anderson et al. 1985).

The level of competition for a hospital is not always apparent. Approximately one-fourth of all hospitals do not have another hospital within 15 miles. Of course, many of these are located in rural areas. In such situations, most physicians admit patients at the only hospital in the area (Luft et al. 1986). Indeed, when more hospitals are available, physicians tend to admit their patients to different hospitals (Luft and Maerki 1985).

Even where other hospitals exist within a 15-mile radius, there may be other factors that limit competition. For example, hospitals located in an ethnic neighborhood of a city may attract patients primarily from that neighborhood. The same differentiation could occur across religious or income levels (Shelton 1989). Patients from other areas, religions, or incomes may be reluctant to use the facility (Anderson et al. 1985). Likewise, hospitals that serve special patients (e.g., Shriners' hospitals, Veterans' hospitals) and county hospitals that only serve the indigent are not really involved in the local hospital market.

In hospital markets where only several hospitals exist, the markets may be more oligopolistic than competitive. In a market with only a few hospitals, each realizes that its pricing actions will affect the prices of its competitors and thus affect the price structure of the entire market. If one hospital gives discounts, for example, all might be forced to follow suit. Thus, after all have reduced prices, each hospital's share of the market might remain essentially the same. The only change would be that all would receive less income for the same services.

As a result of the above dynamics, hospitals in oligopolistic markets often choose to compete in services rather than costs. Hence, each hospital tries to establish a better reputation than another. They often select different areas to emphasize. One might specialize in open-heart surgery, another in a special burn unit, while another might have a state-of-the-art unit for critical newborns.

This competition in services is encouraged by physicians. Since physicians want privileges at hospitals with the latest equipment, hospitals seek the latest technology in order to attract more physicians and their patients. Thus, hospitals, influenced by their medical directors and staffs, attempt to maximize their status relative to competitors. Of course, such competition usually increases costs.

Whenever hospitals engage in quality competition, they are not particularly receptive to courting by HMOs which seek price discounts. In a service-competitive market, HMOs' utilization mechanisms face more resistance from physicians and hospital administrators because neither the buyers nor users of health care services are price-sensitive (Anderson et al. 1985). Hence, HMOs find that marketing their plans to employers and employees is difficult in a service-competitive market. Moreover, a primary goal of most HMOs is to reduce inpatient utilization which runs counter to the primary goal of most hospitals.

Hospitals are expanding their services beyond inpatient care. They are more interested in "vertical integration" of health care in order to control more of the "inputs" which lead to patient hospitalization (Goldsmith 1981). Thus, hospitals diversify into ambulatory care, wellness programs, and outpatient activities to draw referrals into hospitals. Similarly, they may move into long-term or home health care to maintain control over patients after hospitalization (Anderson et al. 1985). Hospitals' involvement in these activities could place them in more direct competition with HMOs who may also have such facilities, and whose main goal in operating them is to keep patients out of the hospital.

Many hospitals' local markets are changing as a result of several factors. Within the last decade, many hospitals' markets have suffered from a surplus of hospital beds. Thus, HMOs which can deliver a large number of patients have become more attractive to hospitals.

Similarly, a physician surplus has developed within the last decade. With a greater number of physicians, hospitals have been less concerned that contracting with an HMO would upset physicians. Likewise, as a result of the greater number of physicians and the higher level of competition among doctors, hospitals have not needed to "court" physicians by providing all of the latest technical advances. Thus, some of the physician pressure for quality competition is being replaced by a greater willingness to engage in price competition.

Employers have grown increasingly concerned about health care costs in the last four years. It is unlikely that they will continue to pay double digit increases for their employees' health care. Most surveys of employers reveal that their main concern is cost containment not quality. As a result, it seems unlikely that employers and other large purchasers of health care will tolerate quality or service competition among hospitals when the result is to further increase costs.

Many hospital markets include a considerable number of competitors. Indeed, approximately 25 percent of all hospitals have eleven or more competitors within a fifteen-mile radius (Luft et al. 1986). With this many competitors, it is difficult for any one hospital to predict the behavior of competitors. Likewise, the actions of any one competitor may not affect the entire market. Therefore, cartels and oligopolies cannot develop as readily in such markets. Moreover, price competition is more likely to develop.

As a result of these recent changes in local hospital markets, more hospitals

are receptive to overtures from HMOs seeking special p
sharing arrangements. At least in theory, there are a nu
HMO could provide a hospital.

## Benefits of HMOs for Hospitals

Theoretically, HMOs could provide a number of be
they could increase the referrals to the hospitals and increase inpatient
They could provide additional opportunity for hospitals to develop ambulatory care programs and wellness programs that in turn could increase inpatient utilization.

Second, HMOs could become political allies of hospitals as they seek clearances from local health systems agencies and could assist the hospital in the development of data and management information systems on patients, providers, and costs and revenues.

Last, but certainly not least, the HMO could eliminate many of the hospitals' collection problems (such as bad debts, late payments, and paperwork (Anderson et al. 1985).

## Types of Contracts Between Hospitals and HMOs

There are a number of payment arrangements between hospitals and HMOs including:

a. Discounts on the billed charges.
b. A global rate in which the hospital agrees to provide all hospital services to an HMO for an agreed upon annual payment per enrollee.
c. An all-inclusive rate per HMO-admitted patient where the hospital agrees to provide all hospital services.
d. All inclusive per diem rates in which the hospital agrees to provide all hospital services (Some contracts exclude very expensive admissions such as cardiac surgery or burn cases. Other contracts may have decreasing per-diem rates as the number of patient days increase.).
e. Hospitals bill their normal charges against a fixed amount based on a capitated charge per HMO enrollee. The hospital may receive full payment for services until the fixed amount is reached. If charges exceed this amount, both the HMO and the hospital may share the costs (Morrisey et al. 1983; Kralewski et al. 1983).
f. Hospitals bill full charges with a ''hold-back'' to cover inpatient expenses beyond a certain amount.

Group-model HMOs tend to negotiate a contract with a single hospital and include other hospitals as their enrollment expands to other areas (Morrisey et al. 1983). Conversely, IPAs tend to use nearly every hospital in a market (Kralewski et al. 1983).

also common for HMOs to sign contracts with different hospitals for erent kinds of services. Thus, an HMO might contract with one hospital for edical/surgical services, with another for obstetrics, and yet another for chemical dependency (Morrisey et al. 1983).

Contracts are initiated by both hospitals and HMOs. Different factors motivate each to seek a contract. An HMO's decision to seek a contract is guided by preexisting ties to a hospital or its medical staff, cost per inpatient day, its reputation and location and its willingness to provide a discount or share risk (Anderson et al. 1985).

A hospital's eagerness to sign a contract with an HMO is dependent on the hospital's present occupancy rate, the potential of the HMO to generate new patients from the HMO, and the potential loss of patients if a contract is not signed. Dollars do not necessarily determine if an HMO and a hospital will sign a contract. A hospital's location and reputation are valuable to an HMO. Likewise, HMOs who have physicians with established admitting privileges are valuable resources to the hospital.

### Factors Limiting HMOs' Influence Over Hospitals

Even though HMOs have potential benefits for hospitals and despite the recent changes in hospitals' local markets that make them more receptive to HMOs, there are numerous factors that limit HMOs' influence over hospitals.

First, it is rare for any single HMO to be able to provide a significant percentage of any single hospital's patients. An HMO membership of 125,000 is needed to completely support a 200-bed hospital (Anderson et al. 1985) Yet only 74 HMOs in the country or 12 percent of all HMOs have more than 100,000 members. Even those HMOs with large memberships may not have these members concentrated in a single hospital market.

Second, HMOs enroll approximately 12 percent of the nation's population, and it is rare for HMOs in any state to enroll more than 25 percent of the population. Moreover, this enrollment is generally split among several HMOs in any geographical area. Thus, few HMOs have sufficient market penetration in a local area to have a sizable impact on a single hospital in the area.

Third, some of an HMO's members will use out-of-plan providers and thus further undermine the HMO's ability to assure a large percentage of the hospital's patients. Thus, an HMO's influence with a hospital is further reduced.

Fourth, as an HMO attracts more members, it generally encompasses a larger geographical area and thus has to have more hospitals in different locations to serve the added members. Paradoxically, the larger an HMO becomes, the more difficult it becomes to channel members to only one or two hospitals. Indeed, one reason for the HMO's growth could be that it has contracted with a number of hospitals rather than only one or two (Shelton 1989).

Fifth, it is not easy for an HMO to move patients from one hospital to another. Even where an HMO has a high percentage of a hospital's census, it is not clear whether the HMO produced this concentration or if it simply recruited physicians and members who used the hospital. Many enrollees have strongly held preferences for a particular hospital and will not easily accept another. Similarly, employers are often hesitant to insist that their employees shift from one hospital to another for fear of antagonizing them.

Sixth, hospitals know that if they give discounts to one HMO, they may have to give similar discounts to other HMOs, PPOs and traditional insurers. Therefore, they may be hesitant to offer any discounts.

Seventh, while HMOs want discounts, they must be concerned about more than just the lowest-price care. They must also be concerned about their patients' and physicians' desires. Likewise, HMOs often seek hospitals for their locational advantages and for their prestige in order to attract both physicians and enrollees into the HMOs.

Eighth, since HMOs use extensive utilization review, they succeed in treating many of their members in outpatient facilities who otherwise might have been hospitalized. As a result, those HMO patients who are hospitalized tend to be sicker than the average inpatient and more expensive for the hospital. Lengths-of-stay for HMO members tend to be longer. Thus, hospitals are hesitant to give discounts from their normal charges to a group whose hospitalization is often more expensive than the average.

Ninth, the fastest growing HMOs in the last few years have been IPAs. Since IPAs are the most decentralized of HMOs, they are the least able to direct patients to any particular hospital.

Tenth, the hospitals with the most incentives to give discounts may be those least attractive to HMOs. Inner-city urban hospitals may seek to attract HMO members, but their facilities and location may not be sufficiently attractive even at a lower price to obtain an HMO contract. Conversely, more prosperous suburban hospitals, while attractive to HMOs, may see little reason to offer discounts.

For all of these reasons, HMOs have not had as much influence on hospitals as might first appear. The chief way that HMOs have realized savings in hospitalization has been by rigorous use of utilization review and by reducing admissions, not by obtaining discounts.

HMOs will have the greatest influence in local markets where:

- HMOs have numerous members,
- One HMO tends to be dominant,
- Hospitals are numerous,
- Physicians are comparatively plentiful,
- Hospital occupancy is low and capacity is high,
- Hospital prices are comparatively high,

- There are large employers with geographically concentrated work forces who are less educated and accustomed to low benefits, low pay or both, and
- Employees are in a highly price-competitive industry (Shelton 1989).

### Ownership of Hospitals and HMOs

Outside of the Kaiser plans, HMOs rarely own hospitals. A 200-bed hospital would need approximately 125,000 HMO members to keep it occupied. Most HMOs have fewer members. Moreover, even if an HMO had sufficient members, the enrollees would need to be concentrated in one local area so that the hospital would be convenient to all. Also, most of the intensive capital expenditures required to construct a hospital are fixed and would be borne by the HMO even if its enrollment declined. Most HMOs prefer the greater financial flexibility provided by contracting for hospital services.

Relatively few HMOs are owned by hospitals. Perhaps a primary reason for this relatively small hospital investment in HMOs is that they basically have contradicting goals. Hospitals want to hospitalize patients, and HMOs want to keep their members out of hospitals.

Hospitals are also weak in the kinds of organizational structure, actuarial abilities, marketing knowledge, and capitalization strength needed by HMOs (Johnson 1981).

## PHARMACIES AND HMOs

Approximately one-fourth of HMOs cover prescription drugs in the basic benefits package. However, three-fourths provide such benefits as a rider (Gold et al. 1989). Most enrollees purchase the rider and almost 90 percent of all HMO members have pharmacy coverage. Virtually all of the plans require a copayment. Most HMOs limit coverage of over-the-counter drugs, experimental drugs and birth control devices (Gold et al. 1989).

One in five HMOs use in-house pharmacies. Three-fourths of all staff-model HMOs and over half of all group-model HMOs have in-house pharmacies (Marion 1990). IPAs and network model HMOs contract almost exclusively with outside pharmacies.

Those HMOs using outside pharmacies tend to contract with retail drug chains. While mail-order drug plans have increased during the last five years, only 8 percent of HMOs used such plans in 1989 (Marion 1990).

Since approximately 10 percent of all HMO expenses are for drugs, HMOs pursue a variety of drug cost-containment practices (Marion 1990). These include copayments, utilization reviews, formularies, and mandatory use of generic drugs.

Nearly all plans require a copayment which averages about three dollars per prescription. Approximately half of all plans have drug utilization reviews. Also, about 40 percent of all HMOs have drug formularies that govern which pharmaceuticals can be prescribed by physicians (Marion 1990). Moreover, about 80 percent of all HMOs require the use of generic drugs when available.

Staff-model HMOs' drug costs, as a percentage of total operating costs, are approximately half those of other HMOs (6 versus 10 percent). The primary reason for these lower costs probably is the staff HMOs' much more aggressive use of in-house pharmacies and formularies.

## CONCLUSION

The increasing supply of physicians should permit most HMOs to recruit physicians more selectively. Thus, HMOs should be able to attract physicians who more nearly agree with an HMO's philosophy and approach to medical care. As a result, HMOs should be more nearly able to obtain the practice styles they desire.

As large employers place additional pressure on HMOs to control costs, HMOs will more aggressively utilize the methods discussed in this chapter to control the behavior of physicians. The increasing competition among doctors will promote greater receptiveness among doctors to HMOs' overtures. These changes plus the growing familiarity with and acceptance of HMOs by the general public and by physicians, suggest that HMOs' future relations with physicians should be better than in past years.

# 7

# HMOs, Medicare, and Medicaid

The costs of Medicare and Medicaid are two of the most rapidly escalating costs of government. They are increasing at even more rapid rates than the health care costs for the general population. As the baby boom ages, the outlook is for even more dramatic increases. Thus, corporations and employees must be concerned about higher taxes to support such increases. HMOs have some potential to ameliorate these increases even while providing quality medical care to the less able portions of our population.

## PROBLEMS OF MEDICARE AND OPPORTUNITIES FOR HMOs

A major problem of Medicare is its fragmented approach to health care delivery. The numerous systems for financing, reimbursing, and delivering care produce a fragmented and patchwork system that is biased towards acute care services and institutionalization (Iversen et al. 1986). Part A of Medicare, which is the hospital insurance, covers hospitalization, short-term, skilled nursing home care, and limited home health care. Part B covers physician and outpatient hospital services. Medicaid covers long-term nursing home care for the elderly once they have "spent down" their own funds for their long-term care expenses.

Over 95 percent of the Medicare budget is spent on hospital and physician services, while less than 10 percent is spent on personal care services such as home health care (Iversen et al. 1986). Thus, Medicare focuses almost entirely on financing acute care services with an emphasis on hospitalization. Likewise, the Medicaid program is also biased toward institutionalization with over two-thirds of all Medicaid expenditures for elderly recipients spent on nursing home care and only 3 percent spent on home health care.

This limited, fragmented coverage is not appropriate for the elderly who have high rates of chronic and multiple illnesses (Iversen et al. 1986). Indeed, over 85 percent of all elderly have some chronic illness. In fact, elderly persons report an average of over four illnesses per year (Bates and Brown 1988). Given this frequency of conditions, the elderly often present an overlap of mental and physical disorders that create problems in detecting, diagnosing, and managing their health care needs.

The illnesses of later life often tend to be chronic ones that are managed rather than cured. Chronic conditions among the elderly require more than just the treatment of medical conditions. Individuals' mobility, social, mental, and emotional conditions can affect their health and functional status. Thus, a variety of different treatments are necessary. Moreover, multiple conditions require integration of numerous health services (Iversen et al. 1986). If services are not coordinated, different treatments could duplicate or adversely affect each other (Iversen et al. 1986).

In general, Medicare and Medicaid are financing mechanisms that are independently designed and managed for acute and institutional care. There is little or no integration between these programs. Medicare pays for some hospitalization, and Medicaid pays for nursing home care. Neither the financing nor the delivery of these programs is coordinated. Even though the nature of elderly health care needs suggests a continuum of integrated medical and supportive services to provide appropriate care and to maintain the independence of the elderly as long as possible, the current public systems do not provide this continuum (Iversen et al. 1986).

The fragmentation in the current programs contributes to confusion. Many elderly do not understand the provisions and rules of Medicare. Moreover, as advanced age occurs and as mental and physical conditions tend to mount, the different programs become even more confusing.

In addition to being fragmented, the current programs are quite costly. Expenditures for Medicare have risen from $35 billion in 1980 to over $100 billion in 1990. Reimbursement per enrollee has also risen dramatically and faster than per capita health care expenditures for the U.S. population.

Medicaid expenditures have escalated at an even more dramatic pace. While Medicaid is often viewed as a health care program for poor families headed by single parents, it also is the primary financing system for long-term nursing care for the elderly. This occurs as the elderly ''spend-down'' their own funds for nursing home care until they become eligible for Medicaid support.

Medicaid expenditures have often escalated at double digit rates. For example, between 1975 and 1985, Medicaid expenditures increased from approximately $12 billion to $40 billion at an average annual increase of 13.6 percent (Iversen et al. 1986). This was 40 percent higher than the general increase in health expenditures. Individuals sixty-five or older generate 40 percent of Medicaid expenditures even though they are only 15 to 17 percent of total Medicaid recipients.

These problems of fragmentation, confusion and high costs within the Medicare system pose at least theoretical opportunities for HMOs in Medicare. In other words, the structure, operations and incentives within HMOs might ameliorate some of the problems faced by the elderly within Medicare and Medicaid.

Medicare uses the fee-for-service system to reimburse most providers of care to the elderly. Thus, Medicare, as with health care in general, suffers from the inflationary effects of the FFS system. The FFS incentives encourage the delivery of more services and the most expensive services. Likewise, under the FFS system, more expensive institutionalization is generally encouraged over less expensive care.

The financial arrangements within most HMOs would appear to reduce costs since doctors in HMOs are either paid on a capitated basis or because they share part of the risk pool. Therefore, if HMOs received a capitation from the government for each elderly enrollee in the HMO, the HMO would have a built-in incentive to control both the utilization and costs of services by their elderly enrollees. Also, an HMO would not seek to institutionalize an elderly enrollee unless this was the only available alternative. Since institutionalization is more expensive, HMOs would probably seek to keep enrollees out of hospitals and nursing homes until absolutely necessary. It would probably be in an HMO's financial self-interest to keep semi-independent elderly in their own homes, as opposed to nursing homes, for as long as possible. Thus, HMOs would have both the structure and financial incentives to provide the continuum of care for the elderly that is often absent in Medicare.

The structure of most HMOs appears, at least in theory, to offer some amelioration of the fragmentation and confusion found within Medicare and Medicaid. HMOs' formal organizational structures tend to promote more peer review and more formal and informal consultation among physicians in the group. Since HMOs provide care through a formally organized effort, they should be better able to integrate the efforts of various providers. Hence, HMOs should be better able to offer the continuity and coordination needed for the chronic care needs of the elderly.

The emphasis on ambulatory care in HMOs could reduce the threat of intrusive practice patterns and excessive hospitalization that could contribute only marginally, if not actually be detrimental, to the diagnosis and management of illness. This may be particularly important when the elderly may not feel capable of exercising much independent judgment concerning the need for hospitalization.

Finally, most HMOs provide more comprehensive care which could be particularly important to the elderly who not only need a greater number and variety of services, but who also may be less capable than the average individual in coordinating care. For example, HMOs often provide some form of wellness programs, prescription services, as well as hearing aids and eyeglasses. Of course, the elderly have greater need for most of these services.

## EARLY HISTORY OF HMOs' INVOLVEMENT IN MEDICARE

Since the enactment of the original Medicare legislation in 1966, Medicare has provided a number of contracting options to HMOs which wanted to participate in Medicare. Initially, contracts were available only for Part B services with Part A payments made directly to hospitals. Reimbursement to HMOs for Part B services were offered as retrospective payments for actual costs or as prospective payments later adjusted for actual costs. Since payments were retrospective, limited to Part B services, and demanded considerable paperwork, most HMOs did not contract with Medicare (Iversen and Polich 1985).

Because of increasing health care costs, the Medicare Act was amended in 1972 to provide more incentives for HMOs to contract with Medicare. These amendments allowed for advance payments to HMOs based on capitated rates for the delivery of both Part A and Part B services. HMOs could enter into either cost or "risk-based" contracts with Medicare for the provision of both Part A and Part B services.

With either risk or cost contracts, reimbursement was provided through monthly capitation payments based on Medicare's estimate of the plan's costs for providing services to its Medicare enrollees. If an HMO chose the cost option, actual costs were calculated at the end of the contract period based on cost reports from the HMO. Prior reimbursements to the plan were then adjusted to reflect allowable and reasonable costs (Langwell and Hadley 1986).

HMOs that chose the risk option had their costs compared to a retrospectively determined adjusted average per capita cost (AAPCC), which represented what Medicare's costs would have been for the enrollees if they had been in the fee-for-service system. The AAPCC was and is adjusted for the age, sex, geographic location, and welfare/institutional status difference between Medicare HMO enrollees and nonenrollees. If actual costs were more than 100 percent of the AAPCC, the HMO was required to absorb all of the loss. On the other hand, if actual costs were less than 100 percent of the AAPCC, the HMO would split the savings equally with the government up to a maximum of 20 percent of the AAPCC (10 percent to the HMO and 10 percent to the government). Any savings beyond 20 percent went entirely to the government.

Since the 1972 amendments limited HMO's savings or profits, but not their risks, the legislation offered few financial incentives to HMOs. As a result, by 1980, 14 years after the introduction of Medicare, only 31 HMOs had cost contracts with Medicare (23,498 enrollees), and only one HMO had a risk contract with Medicare (19,268 enrollees) (Langwell and Hadley 1986). The failure of HMOs to contract with Medicare, particularly on a risk-basis, resulted from Medicare's failure to offer sufficient financial incentives. Moreover, the retrospective cost-based reimbursement system used by Medicare conflicted with HMOs' usual reliance on prospectively determined rates. This reluctance of HMOs to contract with Medicare pointed to the need for a major change in government policy if HMOs were to be more involved in providing health care to the elderly.

## TAX EQUITY AND FISCAL RESPONSIBILITY ACT OF 1982 (TEFRA)

A major change in government policy came with the passage of TEFRA in 1982. Under TEFRA regulations, payment to HMOs is determined using two combined methodologies—the AAPCC and the Adjusted Community Rate (ACR). The ACR is what the HMO's premium would be if it provided its Medicare package to its general non-Medicare membership. This rate is adjusted to reflect the complexity or intensity of services used by the Medicare enrollees.

HMOs receive 95 percent of the AAPCC per each beneficiary. The AAPCC is intended to be the average amount that Medicare would have paid for health care services of HMO Medicare enrollees if they had remained in the FFS system. First, a national Medicare reimbursement average is computed. This figure is multiplied by the ratio of county to national per capita reimbursements for the five most recent years of available data. This figure is then multiplied by a ratio factor that accounts for differences in the HMO enrollees versus the FFS beneficiaries among certain risk classes (age, sex, welfare status, and institutional status). The AAPCC is determined each year by the Health Care Financing Administration (HCFA) which uses national historical data on Medicare expenditures.

HMOs receive 95 percent of the AAPCC as prospective payments. However, if the ACR is less than the AAPCC, the HMO must convert this difference into additional benefits for its Medicare enrollees or reduce the enrollees' premiums.

Although TEFRA made HMOs more available to Medicare beneficiaries, there are numerous issues that affect the potential of HMOs to provide health care to the elderly. These include the benefits and quality of care provided by Medicare HMOs, as well as the costs of such care. Moreover, disagreement over real costs and savings often centers on whether biased selection occurs in Medicare HMOs. Concern about biased selection has prompted numerous suggestions for revising the AAPCC and Medicare's payment methodologies. All of these issues are discussed below.

## BENEFITS PACKAGES IN HMOs CONTRACTING WITH MEDICARE

The Medicare program permits significant out-of-pocket exposure to Medicare beneficiaries. Thus, many elderly purchase at least some supplemental health insurance from traditional health insurers. Such insurance provides some supplemental coverage beyond that which is provided by the standard Medicare package. Since HMOs that contract with Medicare must by law provide the same standard Medicare package, they see the supplemental insurers as the primary competition in the Medicare market.

The first HMOs in the Medicare market were faced with the problems of educating Medicare beneficiaries to the HMO concept and designing benefit packages that would be sufficiently appealing to attract the elderly to a health care financing and delivery system that was new and unfamiliar (Langwell and Hadley 1989). Thus, many Medicare HMOs offered benefit packages considerably more attractive than the standard Medicare Part A and B benefits (Langwell et al. 1987). Some of the added benefits included: reducing the limits, copayments, and deductibles on traditional Medicare coverage, preventive care, extended hospital days, prescriptions, vision and hearing exams, and some mental and dental care (Polich et al. 1987; Brown and Langwell 1988; Bates and Brown 1988; Langwell and Hadley 1989).

It is not clear that these enhanced benefits offered by Medicare HMOs can be sustained over time. HMOs may have been too generous in their initial attempts to attract enrollees. Therefore, they may have to reduce benefits or increase premiums. There is some recent evidence to suggest that both of these trends are occurring (Iversen and Polich 1987; Langwell and Hadley 1989). Nevertheless, benefits provided by Medicare HMOs appear to significantly expand those available under Medicare, and to do so at a price significantly below that offered through traditional supplemental Medicare insurance.

## QUALITY OF CARE IN MEDICARE HMOs

Given the age and more fragile health status of Medicare beneficiaries, the quality of care in Medicare HMOs is a critical issue. As noted in Chapter 4, there are several ways to evaluate quality including access to care, the process of care, and health status or health outcomes. Also, enrollee satisfaction is another indicator of quality.

One aspect of quality is access to care. Of course, there is some fear that HMOs might try to control utilization by creating obstacles to care (e.g., long waiting times, use of gatekeepers, prior authorization requirements). However, recent research on Medicare HMOs indicates that both HMO enrollees and fee-for-service enrollees report similar high rates of provider follow-up for urgent, semi-urgent and nonurgent symptoms (Langwell and Hadley 1989).

It should be remembered that Medicare HMOs often offer a large number of services not available in basic Medicare. This fact combined with the knowledge that many HMO Medicare enrollees (approximately 36 percent) did not have Medicare supplemental insurance before they joined an HMO, indicates that HMOs expanded at least potential access to more services (Brown and Langwell 1988). Moreover, very few enrollees had prior coverage for services not covered by Medicare supplemental insurance but often provided by Medicare HMOs including dental services, nursing and home aide care, eyeglasses, and prescription drugs (Brown and Langwell 1988).

In terms of process measures of quality, research also indicates that Medicare HMO providers obtained better medical histories, gave more complete physical examinations, ordered more screening tests, and used a greater frequency of immunizations than did FFS Medicare providers (Langwell and Hadley 1989). The same research indicates that HMOs and fee-for-service doctors do equally well in terms of follow-up on abnormal test results or the detection of serious illness. Likewise, both FFS and HMO Medicare doctors managed diabetes mellitus in very similar ways. In the treatment of hypertensives, however, HMO providers were more likely to document medical history taking, physical exams and interventions (Langwell and Hadley 1989).

In comparisons of Medicare patients in HMOs and in the fee-for-service system who had congestive heart failure (CHF) and colorectal cancer (CRC), no significant differences were found between the two groups in terms of inpatient management of CHF or in prescribing and monitoring therapies for CHF. However, HMO doctors were much more likely to schedule follow-up visits within one week of discharge more frequently than FFS doctors (Langwell and Hadley 1989).

In the first evaluation of CRC patients, HMO doctors were more likely than their FFS colleagues to document history taking and to perform an endoscopic or radiologic procedure (Langwell and Hadley 1989). There were no significant differences between the two groups regarding the stage of cancer at the time of diagnosis or operative procedure.

Langwell and Hadley (1989) also compared health status of Medicare beneficiaries in the FFS system and in Medicare HMOs. They found no significant differences between the two groups in the percent of beneficiaries whose health status declined between the baseline and follow-up surveys and no significant differences in the percent who showed no change in health status.

## SATISFACTION OF MEDICARE BENEFICIARIES IN HMOs

Another way to evaluate the quality of care in Medicare HMOs is to examine the satisfaction of Medicare HMO enrollees with their care. Apparently, most are very satisfied with their care. A Kaiser Permanente survey indicated that 92 percent of the Medicare enrollees were satisfied with the HMO, while only 2 percent were dissatisfied. Approximately 84 percent believed that their doctor was "as good or better than other doctors," and less than 5 percent rated overall access to care as dissatisfactory ("HMO/Medicare Demonstration Projects" 1985).

Langwell and Hadley (1989) found that 81 percent of HMO Medicare enrollees were "very satisfied." This result was essentially the same percentage as for Medicare patients in FFS settings. While the overall satisfaction level of both groups were similar, they differed on specific dimensions or components of overall satisfaction. Nonenrollees were more satisfied with the professional competence of their doctors and their willingness to discuss problems. On the other hand, HMO enrollees were more satisfied with waiting time for an appointment and opportunity to see a doctor. Also, HMO enrollees were much more satisfied with the time and effort required to process claims. Most HMOs eliminate or minimize claims processing for enrollees, and this apparently contributes significantly to overall satisfaction levels (Langwell and Hadley 1989).

Another way of measuring satisfaction is to compare HMO Medicare enrollees' level of satisfaction with care in the HMO to the care they received before joining an HMO. Langwell and Hadley (1989) found that only 64 percent of enrollees reported being very satisfied with their FFS care compared to 81 percent who were very satisfied with the HMO care. Moreover, 29 percent of enrollees reported greater satisfaction with their HMO care than with care from FFS providers. Conversely, only 9 percent reported a decrease in satisfaction. These results indicate that Medicare beneficiaries who join and remain in a Medicare HMO increase their level of satisfaction with medical care and are as satisfied with care as are those elderly who remain in the FFS sector (Langwell and Hadley 1989).

Of course, these satisfaction surveys did not include those who had disenrolled from the HMOs. Thus, disenrollment, particularly disenrollment that is not a result of moving, is significant in determining satisfaction of enrollees.

Group Health Association demonstration projects reported a 1 to 5 percent disenrollment rate; however, less than 2 percent of this was attributed to client dissatisfaction (''HMO/Medicare Demonstration Projects'' 1985). Similarly, Kaiser Permanente experienced less than 5 percent disenrollment during the first year of its HMO/Medicare project (''Survey Finds Elderly Highly Satisfied'' 1984).

Langwell and Hadley (1989) found that 15 percent of enrollees in Medicare HMOs disenrolled; however, 25 percent of this group subsequently joined another HMO. Hence, disenrollment tended to be highest in areas with more HMOs. Thus, these particular disenrollees apparently were dissatisfied with a specific HMO but not the HMO concept. They were simply ''shopping around'' for a more attractive HMO plan. If this group is removed, a little more than 10 percent of the enrollees returned to the FFS sector.

All of these disenrollment rates appear low and thus indicate overall general satisfaction. Nevertheless, the reasons for leaving do shed additional light on possible problems within Medicare HMOs. A major complaint of most disenrollees concerned choice of physician. Many who disenrolled within one year of joining said they misunderstood the terms of HMO membership. Numerous disenrollees left because the HMO was not conveniently located.

Bates and Brown (1988) found that the ''old-old'' (e.g., those over eighty) are more likely to disenroll from a Medicare HMO. As the need for long-term care increases with age, the emphasis on ambulatory care by HMOs apparently is less attractive to the ''frail elderly.''

It should be noted that much of the recent research on satisfaction and disenrollment in Medicare HMOs covers the first few years in which the HMOs had TEFRA risk contracts. Part of the overall high satisfaction may reflect the rather generous packages that HMOs designed to attract new enrollees from the FFS sector. If these programs become less generous, satisfaction may obviously decline.

## UTILIZATION AND BIASED SELECTION IN MEDICARE HMOs

There has been relatively little research on utilization in Medicare HMOs. However, research on utilization in HMOs in general (see Chapter 3) indicates that HMOs have reduced hospitalization but that their impact on ambulatory utilization is mixed. This may result from HMOs substituting outpatient care for hospitalization. The limited research on Medicare HMOs indicates that they too decrease hospitalization. Nelson and others (1986) found that hospitalization was considerably lower in Medicare HMOs than for Medicare beneficiaries in the same local market areas who received care in the FFS sector.

Langwell and Hadley (1989) found that Medicare HMOs had reduced hospitalization over a two-year period by approximately 8 percent per year. The lower utilization was the result of lower admission rates rather than shorter lengths of stay. This research also indicated that the HMOs' use of a skilled nursing facility (SNF) increased dramatically. Apparently, the HMOs were replacing hospital days with less expensive SNF days. Langwell and Hadley (1989) were unable to analyze the utilization of ambulatory services.

From this limited research and other more general research on utilization in HMOs, it appears that Medicare HMOs probably do reduce hospital utilization. However, their impact on overall health care utilization is much less clear and more research is needed in this area.

This reduction in utilization could result from more efficient utilization review in Medicare HMOs or it could simply be the result of biased selection. As was noted in Chapter 3, biased selection can help or hurt an HMO. If HMOs attract a disproportionately unhealthy portion of the Medicare population (adverse selection), they will suffer economic losses and may eventually have to cancel their contracts. When an HMO cancels its contract, its enrollees must find another plan and thus will suffer some discontinuity of care.

On the other hand, if HMOs attract a disproportionately healthier segment of the Medicare population, the HMO and the Medicare beneficiaries will profit from this "favorable selection." However, the government will be spending more money than it would have spent if the HMO option had not been available and the beneficiaries had continued to receive care in the FFS sector.

Moreover, if there is favorable selection into HMOs, the AAPCC would increase over time. This would occur because average Medicare FFS costs would increase as the low-cost beneficiaries joined HMOs thus leaving the more expensive (i.e., sicker) beneficiaries in the FFS sector. In turn, the amount paid to the Medicare HMOs (95 percent of AAPCC) would increase resulting in even greater expenditures for the Medicare program (Anderson and others 1986). Therefore, the issue of biased selection (adverse or favorable) is of utmost importance when deciding the appropriate pricing or payment method for Medicare beneficiaries in HMOs.

Most studies have revealed favorable selection of Medicare beneficiaries into HMOs. Eggers (1980) and Eggers and Prihoda (1982) found that total Medicare reimbursements over a four-year pre-enrollment period were substantially lower for HMO enrollees in all three HMOs they studied. Moreover, McCall and Wai (1981) and Anderson and Knickman (1984) found that heavy users of Medicare service in one year are much more likely to be heavy users in subsequent years. Thus, if pre-enrollment utilization is low, post-enrollment utilization is also likely to be low.

Langwell and Hadley (1989) in their analysis of 26 Medicare HMOs found that Medicare enrollees tended to be younger and in excellent self-reported health, while nonenrollees were more likely to be in nursing homes, seeing a regular physician, aware of a health problem that they thought might require hospitalization, and had more out-of-pocket expenditures for health care in the previous year.

Langwell and Hadley (1989) also found that the average total Medicare reimbursements per enrollee across all HMOs were 21 percent below the AAPCC-adjusted average reimbursements for nonenrollees. Thus, the enrollees were much less likely to utilize health care services prior to enrolling in an HMO.

Of course, disenrollees from Medicare HMOs can also produce biased selection if disproportionately healthier or sicker enrollees tend to leave Medicare HMOs. Disenrollment could be particularly significant because beneficiaries can disenroll and enroll in another plan at any time where most non-Medicare HMO enrollees can change plans only once per year.

Research indicates that disenrollees from Medicare HMOs tend to be in worse health and have a higher propensity to use health services than those Medicare beneficiaries who remain in the HMO (Langwell and Hadley 1989; Bates and Brown 1988). Since one percent of the population accounts for one-quarter of the medical expenditures, and since the very old tend to be in this one percent and are also likely to leave HMOs, one can see that HMO encouraged disenrollment in just a few cases could be significant financially (Bates and Brown 1988).

In light of this concern about biased selection, it is well to remember that Welch (1985), and Riley and others (1989) found that regression toward the mean occurs over time with both high and low users of care moving toward the average. Thus, the differences in prior utilization between enrollees and nonenrollees may overstate the effect of favorable selection on future utilization.

## MODIFICATIONS OF THE AAPCC

Biased selection would not be a problem if the AAPCC considered and incorporated factors that most contribute to the bias. In other words, if the AAPCC in determining payments for Medicare beneficiaries in HMOs compensated for those factors that most affect bias or ''predict'' subsequent utilization, then favorable or adverse selection would not be financially significant. If the appropriate predictive factors were used, then biased selection would not matter because the rates would be based on accurate predictions of future utilization.

There is considerable research which indicates that the AAPCC is a poor predictor of both utilization and health care expenditures (Eggers and Prihoda 1982; Anderson et al. 1983; Hornbrook 1984; Beebe et al. 1985; Langwell and Hadley 1989). These studies suggest that additional factors should be included in the calculation of the AAPCC.

A frequently mentioned modification of the AAPCC is to include prior utilization information in addition to demographic adjustments in the AAPCC. A number of studies have found that prior utilization is a better predictor of future utilization than are demographic variables (McCall and Wai 1981; Anderson and Knickman 1984; Lubitz et al. 1985).

However, there are problems in using prior utilization in the AAPCC. Using prior utilization would reward the inefficient providers or those least able to control utilization. Since many medical decisions are made at the margin, a patient who is not very sick may be kept out of a hospital if there is no adjustment for prior utilization, but may be sent to the hospital if there is adjustment (Newhouse 1986). Thus, an adjustment for prior utilization could create perverse economic incentives.

Another problem in using prior utilization data is that no information would be available on beneficiaries at the time they initially are entitled to Medicare. It would also require HMOs to change their data systems and keep much better records of utilization by each enrollee.

Some have suggested that if prior utilization information was used only for chronic versus self-limiting conditions, and for those conditions that involve minimal versus substantial physician discretion in the decision to hospitalize, then HMOs would have less opportunity to manipulate utilization data in their effort to influence future rates. For example, a self-limiting condition such as cataract removal would not be included because it would not be a good predictor of future use. However, heart disease or chronic uremia would be much better predictors of future use and costs (Anderson and Steinberg 1985).

Others have suggested that information on health status be used to supplement the AAPCC (Thomas et al. 1983; McClure 1984; Lichtenstein and Thomas 1987). As with prior utilization data, there are also problems using health status as a predictor. There is no consensus about the best, most valid measure of health status (Anderson et al. 1986). Moreover, patients with the same condition, but with different levels of severity would produce different utilization and costs (Newhouse 1986). Thus, in addition to condition, level of severity data would be necessary. Moreover, individuals having multiple, compounding conditions (e.g., an individual with diabetes, hypertension, and congestive heart failure) would demand more treatment than indicated by adjustments for the three conditions separately.

Self-reported health status could be manipulated by both patients and doctors who would have a self-interest in reporting the patient's condition as poor. Even if the appropriate risk factors could be incorporated into the AAPCC, they might not be sufficient to significantly reduce Medicare HMO selection bias if HMOs' marketing activities and enrollment strategies promote selection bias. If HMOs can promote favorable bias, they might subvert any refinements in the AAPCC. Therefore, some have proposed that instead of individual HMOs doing their individual marketing, all enrollment functions and marketing activities should be centralized in a broker who would have no self-interest in encouraging favorable selection into any particular HMO. An independent broker agency could provide more objective information about the pros and cons of HMO enrollment than could HMO marketers directly employed by an HMO. Moreover, an independent broker could provide information about the differences among competing HMOs. In theory, an independent broker would have little reason to discourage the enrollment of high-risk beneficiaries.

The Health Care Financing Administration (HCFA) sponsored a three-year demonstration of the HMO broker model in Portland, Oregon. Unfortunately, the results from that demonstration revealed that the broker did not significantly reduce the extent of favorable selection into the Medicare HMOs (Powell and Turner 1990). Of course, the demonstration could have been compromised by the fact that the broker was paid by the HMOs according to the number of beneficiaries enrolled. Thus, there would have been little incentive for an HMO to continue a contract with a broker who increased enrollment of the frail elderly. If there is any chance of the broker model working, the broker should probably be paid by the HCFA on an enrollment basis from dues assessed against participating HMOs who cannot individually market their own plans.

## OTHER PROBLEMS IN MEDICARE-REIMBURSEMENT RATES

In addition to the dispute over selection bias and the capacity of the AAPCC to compensate for it, there have been other reimbursement problems. Rates can vary significantly by county of residence. Thus, there can be dramatic discrepancies in payments for two enrollees in the same HMO with identical utilization who happen to live in adjoining counties even though the HMO's costs for each one are equal (Polich et al. 1987a). This is particularly a problem where rural counties adjoin urban counties. Then most of the medical care for the rural beneficiaries are received in the higher-cost urban county, yet the HMO receives payment rates based on the lower costs of the beneficiary's rural residence.

In order to correct this problem and others associated with the use of county data in the AAPCC, other geographical configurations as a basis for payment have been suggested such as five-digit and three-digit zip code areas. However, recent research indicates that no geographical alternative to counties performed significantly better or worse on measures of homogeneity and stability (Porell et al. 1990).

Another problem with the AAPCC is that areas with low utilization receive a low AAPCC. The idea behind giving HMOs 95 percent of the AAPCC was that HMOs would reduce utilization by being more efficient. However, in areas that are already efficient, HMOs may not be able to offer care at 95 percent of an already low base rate. Therefore, HMOs often avoid signing risk contracts in areas with low FFS utilization and low AAPCC (Polich et al. 1987b).

A third problem is that the AAPCC is based upon Medicare reimbursement in an area, not the actual cost of providing medical care. Thus, the base on which the AAPCC is calculated is inadequate in that it does not include out-of-pocket costs by Medicare beneficiaries and non-Medicare covered services. This could be a problem in areas where a high percent of Medicare enrollees are in a Medicare HMO and relatively few in the FFS sector. Likewise, it would be a problem in an area where a high percentage of the Medicare population has access to other types of service (i.e., an area with a large VA hospital or facility).

A fourth problem is that the AAPCC for some rural counties is very low. This could be the result of very efficient medical care delivery in such areas. The more likely case, however, is that such counties have an inadequate supply of providers and reduced access to care. Thus, the low AAPCC could discourage HMOs from offering care in areas most in need of care. Also, if HMOs did contract with Medicare in such areas, it is very likely that they would experience, particularly at first, high levels of utilization because of past unmet needs. Thus, even while Medicare HMOs in rural areas might experience high utilization, they would be confronted with very low AAPCC reimbursement rates. This is a sure formula to discourage the development of Medicare HMOs in rural areas.

Finally, Medicare HMOs do not receive extra payments for catastrophic cases that are much more expensive. Moreover, it is difficult for HMOs to obtain reinsurance to cover such cases. This can be particularly problematic for new HMOs or HMOs with a relatively small enrollment.

## LONG-TERM CARE AND MEDICARE HMOs

It was noted earlier that one of the major problems of Medicare is that it concentrates almost all expenditures on hospital and physician services. Thus, it concentrates heavily on financing acute care services with an emphasis on hospitalization. Likewise, Medicaid focuses on institutional (nursing home) care.

Since over 80 percent of all elderly have some chronic illness, the emphasis of Medicare and Medicaid on acute, institutionalized care seems incomplete. While chronic conditions are limiting, they often do not require institutional care. It was hoped that Medicare HMOs might provide such care. Yet, this potential has not been realized because HMOs remain essentially acute care providers.

On the one hand, it appears that HMOs would be eager to use home health care as a lower-cost alternative to more expensive hospital care. However, home health care is also an alternative to long-term nursing home care. The Medicare HMO is not responsible for long-term nursing home care. This is financed most often by Medicaid. Thus, it has no incentive to offer a lower-cost home care alternative. Most Medicare HMOs exclude custodial care and home-based supportive services.

HMOs are fearful that if they offered home care services, many of the frail elderly who represent the most expensive cases would be attracted to the HMOs in order to avoid going to a nursing home. Thus, such HMOs would experience adverse selection and not be able to break even or make a profit.

If HMOs offered long-term care, they would be susceptible to "moral hazard" (i.e., insurance-induced demand). Thus, people who were surviving at home alone or with the help of family members would opt for more expensive alternatives if insurance provided such coverage. Hence, insurance would increase total demand.

There are two primary ways to control insurance driven demand. The first is to cover only services that are sufficiently undesirable that only the truly ill would use them (e.g., nursing home care). The second is to have objective criteria of needs that can be easily measured by a physician (Iversen and Polich 1985). However, these controls are very difficult to implement in home health care. Home care programs might replace family and other private care causing large increases in costs.

The federal government has attempted to explore a solution to the long-term care problem through the social health maintenance organization (SHMO) demonstration projects. These efforts attempt to expand coverage of community and nursing home care in a controlled manner and to link this expanded care with a complete acute care system (Greenberg et al. 1988).

SHMOs are financed on a prepaid, capitated, at-risk basis. Medicare beneficiaries voluntarily join the SHMO. It is financed by (1) Medicare which pays 100% of the expected costs in the local area, (2) Medicaid funds, and (3) higher beneficiary premiums. These projects had early problems in attracting sufficient beneficiaries. On the other hand, they had to use a queue system to avoid a high proportion of severely impaired members (Greenberg et al. 1988). There is insufficient information to conclude whether demonstrations should be expanded to the larger population (Newcomer et al. 1990).

## IMPACT OF MEDICARE HMOs

After TEFRA became effective in 1985, the number of Medicare HMOs and Medicare enrollment in HMOs increased dramatically over the next year. Beginning in 1987, however, growth began to slow and started to decline in 1988. In late 1990, just over 1,200,000 Medicare enrollees were in 96 HMOs.

The Medicare HMOs that have been least successful financially are usually younger IPAs with a comparatively small total enrollment (Medicare and non-Medicare) who pay their physicians on a fee-for-service basis, and who are located in areas with relatively low AAPCC levels (Langwell and Hadley 1990).

Thus, those HMOs most likely to be successful are those HMOs that have been operational for many years, and which have extensive managed care experience as well as some experience with older enrollees.

It is apparent that Medicare risk contracting with HMOs generates high levels of satisfaction among Medicare beneficiaries who join and remain in HMOs. Furthermore, they have improved financial access to care for low-income Medicare beneficiaries who are not eligible for Medicaid. In addition, they have provided access to care and quality of care that at least equals if not exceeds that provided by the FFS sector (Langwell and Hadley 1990).

Many beneficiaries who join HMOs have low incomes and did not have a regular source of care before joining an HMO. The unmet needs of these beneficiaries may increase utilization during the first year of enrollment. However, in general most Medicare HMOs experience favorable selection. Once these favorable selection effects are accounted for, it appears that HMOs have only a small effect on hospital use by Medicare beneficiaries (Langwell and Hadley 1990).

The impact of favorable selection indicates that changes are probably needed in the AAPCC payment methodology. It is estimated that HCFA paid between 15 and 33 percent more for beneficiaries enrolled under risk contracts than would have been paid for the individuals in the FFS sector (Langwell and Hadley 1990).

Even though most Medicare HMOs have experienced favorable selection, HMOs are not rushing forward to contract with Medicare. A partial explanation of this reluctance is that it is difficult to predict Medicare risks. Just a few, very expensive cases can eliminate all profits in a Medicare HMO, particularly a small one. Of course, such cases are more likely to be present in the elderly population.

A second reason for the reluctance of HMOs to enter the Medicare market is the comparative difficulty in marketing an HMO to an elderly population. HMOs are often accustomed to marketing to employers who in turn help explain or present the HMO option to their employees. It is much more difficult to appeal to single, isolated individuals. It is even more difficult to market HMOs to elderly individuals who may believe that Medicare already covers all things offered by an HMO, and who may know very little about the HMO concept. Hence, they may not be a particularly receptive group.

If Medicare HMOs that have financial problems cease contracting with Medicare, then it is more and more likely that the remaining Medicare HMOs will experience favorable selection. Because of this skewed participation by HMOs, the overall Medicare payment is likely to be greater than what it would have been in the absence of the HMO enrollments (Wallack et al. 1988). Therefore, it is important that the federal government give more attention to the methods and process of reimbursing Medicare HMOs.

## MEDICAID AND HMOs

As with Medicare, the Medicaid program has numerous problems that HMOs might ameliorate, including:

- high costs as a result of excessive hospitalization, too many tests and prescriptions, unnecessary office visits, and use of expensive hospital emergency rooms for routine care,
- lack of access to primary care in many areas,
- lack of continuity of care,
- lack of preventive services (Freund and Neuschler 1986).

HMOs have been suggested as a way to provide coordinated primary care that could reduce unnecessary and inappropriate emergency room care as well as excessive prescriptions and tests.

HMOs would provide enrollees with a specified benefits package in exchange for a fixed capitation from the state. In theory, this prepayment of a predictable amount would eliminate the state's need to process and pay for individual claims for each service provided to Medicaid recipients. In addition, Medicaid's budget is more predictable since the total payment is established in advance through the per capita payments. Moreover, the state need not be engaged in as much monitoring because this responsibility is shifted to the HMOs which accept the financial risk for their enrollees (DesHarnais 1985).

## HISTORY OF MEDICAID HMOs

Enrolling Medicaid beneficiaries in HMOs was first tried in the early 1970s. In 1972, California contracted with HMOs for comprehensive care of its Medicaid population. While the program was not mandatory, it did encourage Medicaid recipients to enroll in HMOs by imposing copayment requirements on enrollees remaining in the FFS sector.

The number of plans and enrollment grew rapidly. However, California had no criteria for contracts, did not monitor quality and incorrectly estimated payment rates (Welch and Miller 1988). In addition, consumers complained about unethical marketing tactics and denial of care. The California Medicaid HMOs had excessive administrative costs and profits, did not keep utilization records and failed to establish grievance and disenrollment procedures (Welch and Miller 1989).

This early scandalous behavior in California Medicaid HMOs affected national policy. As result, HMOs were not seriously considered until 1981 when Congress passed the Omnibus Budget Reconciliation Act (OBRA). States were permitted to establish their own qualification standards for HMOs serving Medicaid patients and were permitted to have up to 75 percent Medicaid enrollment (up from a previous maximum of 50 percent). Moreover, waivers were permitted that allowed states to limit freedom of choice of providers and variance in the services provided to beneficiaries.

The OBRA gave states the authority to keep beneficiaries in Medicaid HMOs for up to six months after the recipients were no longer eligible for Medicaid

(Oberg et al. 1987). Before this change, HMOs were hesitant to enroll Medicaid recipients because it was not clear how long they would be eligible for Medicaid. The change provided greater stability of Medicaid enrollment in HMOs. One of the difficulties Medicaid HMOs have is their high turnover rates caused by loss of Medicaid eligibility and from voluntary disenrollment (Freund and Neuschler 1986). This high turnover means that Medicaid HMOs must be engaged in continuous and vigorous marketing to keep their Medicaid enrollment from declining.

The OBRA encouraged a great deal of experimentation. While OBRA did not produce large-scale enrollment in HMOs, it did show that HMOs could be used to deliver Medicaid. Most of Medicaid HMO enrollees are found in the West and Midwest and are in older and larger HMOs.

Increasing Medicaid voluntary enrollment is difficult because most Medicaid recipients lack tangible incentives to join HMOs. State Medicaid benefits are often generous, and thus it is hard for HMOs to offer more services as an inducement to enroll. Similarly, since recipients do not pay any premium for their coverage, HMOs cannot attract them with lower out-of-pocket premium payments. As a result, in most metropolitan areas that have voluntary enrollment of Medicaid recipients in HMOs, less than 20 percent, and often less than 10 percent of the total eligibles participate in HMOs (Welch and Miller 1988).

States sometimes offer six months or more of guaranteed eligibility to Medicaid recipients who enroll in an HMO and who agree to remain enrolled for the entire guaranteed period. This is one of the few incentives states have available to encourage Medicaid recipients to voluntarily join HMOs (Freund and Neuschler 1986).

Because of the difficulties in attracting voluntary enrollment in Medicaid HMOs, a number of states have used waivers to establish mandatory HMO enrollment in at least part of the state (Welch and Miller 1988). Thus, there are two distinct alternatives for participation by Medicaid beneficiaries in HMOs: voluntary and mandatory enrollment.

## UTILIZATION AND COSTS OF MEDICAID HMOs

In general, research results from Medicaid HMOs show some lowering of utilization, particularly in emergency room use (Freund et al. 1989). However, it should be noted that inpatient utilization did not decline in Medicaid HMOs as much as it generally does when non-Medicaid enrollees join HMOs.

There is no clear indication that the lower utilization resulted in large cost savings (Freund et al. 1989). Capitation appeared to encourage providers to change their practice patterns, particularly in the use of emergency room use and for specialist care. However, the Medicaid rate setting process for HMOs (which is based on FFS expenditures from prior years) and more utilization review in the FFS sector have resulted in lower cost savings than expected. The fact that many Medicaid HMOs did not significantly reduce inpatient utilization may help explain why costs did not decline as much as expected.

## ACCESS TO CARE IN MEDICAID HMOs

Access is of particular concern in Medicaid HMOs in that the poor may not have the resources of more affluent enrollees to demand care. Freund et al. (1989) found that access of Medicaid HMO enrollees was as good if not better than the access to care of Medicaid recipients in the FFS sector.

Likewise, McCall et al. (1989) found that access to urgent care and routine care was about the same for Medicaid recipients in HMOs and in the FFS sector. However, they did find that HMO enrollees did have less access to emergency room care. However, one should remember that Medicaid recipients often abuse emergency room use when they use it for nonemergency routine health care. Thus, if HMOs make a concerted effort to change this behavior, there will be reduced access.

## QUALITY OF CARE IN MEDICAID HMOs

Quality measures of care in Medicaid HMOs are somewhat mixed. In an analysis of the Rand Health Insurance Experiment data, Ware et al. (1986) found that the health status of low-income participants in the HMO declined in comparison to low-income individuals in the FFS sector. However, Sloss et al. (1987), who also reviewed the Rand Experiment data, found no significant differences in health status among low-income enrollees in HMOs and in the FFS sector.

Freund et al. (1989) found that Medicaid HMO enrollees had the same level of self-assessed health status as those in the FFS sector. However, they also found inadequate care was given by HMOs in several areas including prenatal care and immunization of children.

## SATISFACTION WITH CARE IN MEDICAID HMOs

Most studies of the satisfaction of Medicaid recipients in both HMOs and the FFS system have found that the HMO enrollees are less satisfied with care (Freund et al. 1989; McCall et al. 1989). However, while the levels of satisfaction were lower than for comparison groups in the FFS sector, they were still high. Moreover, most of the Medicaid HMO enrollees in the research studies were required to change providers and systems when they joined an HMO. On the other hand, those remaining in the FFS sector did not have to make any changes. Thus, it is not too surprising that the satisfaction of HMO Medicaid recipients is lower than their counterparts in the FFS sector.

## FUTURE OF MEDICAID HMOs

Most of the research on Medicaid HMOs noted in previous sections indicates that HMOs can lower utilization while maintaining high quality care. Moreover, most Medicaid recipients are relatively satisfied with their care in HMOs. Also, HMOs have the potential to reduce Medicaid costs providing that the states give more attention to appropriate rate-setting.

Yet the potential of HMOs for reducing Medicaid costs will probably not be realized as long as enrollment of Medicaid recipients in HMOs is voluntary. There are simply insufficient incentives for most recipients to enroll. Thus, mandatory enrollment will be necessary if HMOs' full potential is to be realized by Medicaid.

Mandatory enrollment raises concerns about access to care and quality of care. However, much of the research on Medicaid HMOs involved mandatory enrollment, and most of this research indicated no significant problems of access or quality. Moreover, mandatory enrollment does not forbid all choice of providers; rather it eliminates the recipient's choice of reimbursement system. As more and more physicians contract with one or more HMOs, and as HMOs' market shares increase, mandatory enrollment will still provide considerable freedom-of-choice of providers to Medicaid recipients.

Mandatory enrollment will also eliminate any concern about biased selection into HMOs, at least from the perspective of the state versus HMOs. Obviously, there could still be biased selection among competing HMOs even under a mandatory system.

Given the concerns about quality of care under a mandatory system, it is important that any such program have an effective quality assurance program, an effective and well-publicized grievance process, and it should provide an opportunity to disenroll for cause.

## CONCLUSION

We have seen that HMOs have considerable potential to control Medicare and Medicaid costs while also delivering quality care. Moreover, most Medicare and Medicaid beneficiaries in HMOs are reasonably satisfied with access to and quality of care. Yet, unless dramatic steps are taken by the federal government, the full potential of HMOs in Medicare and Medicaid will not be realized.

First, the federal government should consider combining that portion of Medicaid funds that is used for the elderly (primarily for nursing home care) with Medicare. This is the first step in creating a more cohesive system that could respond to the full range or continuum of care needed by the elderly.

Next, the government should consider the mandatory capitation of all Medicare and Medicaid benefits. Such a system should incorporate the appropriate provider risk-sharing incentives to control utilization and costs. Moreover, mandatory capitation would eliminate concerns about biased selection.

With mandatory coverage, the government should give much more attention to the rate-setting and reimbursement system to assure that rates better reflect actual health care costs and utilization. Even in a mandatory system, certain providers would by design or chance enroll a disproportionate share of healthy or unhealthy providers. Providers and the government must be protected against such bias.

Under such a system, the government should require a standard package of benefits that would be uniform across all plans. Optional add-ons could be purchased by beneficiaries. Moreover, the government might consider the use of neutral brokers who would be responsible for the marketing of all plans and the enrollment of Medicare and Medicaid recipients in all plans. One broker would serve each geographical region or area and oversee an annual open enrollment. In addition, the broker would provide non-biased comparative information on the available HMOs to beneficiaries. Such brokers might be paid by the government from assessments levied on HMOs based on the number of their Medicare and Medicaid enrollees. Such a system would tend to reduce the ability of HMOs to use marketing tactics to attract disproportionately healthy individuals.

With mandatory coverage, the government must do much more to assure that quality assurances are present in all contracting plans. Specific criteria must be developed for all HMOs and the government must develop a monitoring process to oversee HMOs' quality assurance procedures. In addition, grievance procedures must exist and be well-publicized in all plans.

The present ability of beneficiaries to disenroll within 30 days of joining an HMO invites instability, inaccurate records, ''doctor shopping'' and greater costs. This should be replaced with the annual lock-in that has proved itself for over forty years in the private sector (Enthoven 1988). The government should closely monitor disenrollments for any information concerning both quality and any HMO attempts to encourage disenrollment of high-risk members.

Perhaps the biggest fear of mandatory capitation is concern about beneficiaries' loss of freedom to select providers. Of course, beneficiaries would select HMOs or other capitated plans as well as individual providers within the competing plans. The major loss of freedom would be the use of fee-for-service reimbursement. With mandatory coverage, more plans would be developed and many more providers would be attracted to capitated reimbursement. Thus, there should be ample providers for beneficiaries to select from.

While these suggestions may at first appear extreme, without such changes, HMOs will continue to be little used by Medicare and Medicaid recipients, and their potential to control costs while also integrating care will not be realized.

# 8

# HMOs in Rural Areas

Rural areas are not generally viewed as fertile ground for the development of HMOs because the population is too sparse, the physicians are too opposed, or because no financing can be found. Yet, such areas are often those most in need of effective and efficient medical care. Moreover, there are thousands of employers in rural areas who might want an HMO option. For example, rural areas are home to more than twenty Fortune 1000 companies that employ thousands of workers in manufacturing, forestry and mining industries (Van Hook 1988).

## HEALTH PROBLEMS IN RURAL AREAS

Rural areas often have more pronounced health problems than urban centers. While these problems often deter HMO development, they paradoxically also point to the need for the integrated systems of care available in HMOs.

Most evidence suggests that rural residents have more serious and severe health problems than do their urban counterparts. Rural residents tend to have a greater incidence of chronic illnesses such as arthritis, visual and hearing impairments, thyroid and kidney problems, heart disease, hypertension, and emphysema (National Center for Health Statistics 1986).

The greater extent of chronic illnesses may be explained in part by the higher proportion of elderly in rural populations. Often the younger individuals leave the rural community in search of employment and steady income. The chronic illnesses may also be explained by the lack of adequate care plus the typically demanding occupations of rural areas.

Rural residents are more likely to be uninsured than are urban residents (17 versus 14 percent), and the gap is widest at the lowest-income levels (Hartwell 1988). This probably results from the employment of most rural residents in agriculture or small businesses which are less likely to provide health insurance to their employees. In addition, incomes are lower in rural areas, and residents are less able to afford insurance when it is not provided by their employers.

Medicaid coverage is less likely to be available to rural poor. This results from several factors. First, Medicaid assistance has been more generous in the heavily urbanized, less rural states. Second, Medicaid eligibility favors the single-parent household which is more prevalent in urban areas. There may be greater cultural resistance in urban areas to enrolling in welfare programs. Finally, many rural poor or their physicians may simply be unfamiliar with Medicaid (Hartwell 1988).

Despite the apparent greater need for health care among rural residents, there is a shortage of providers in rural areas. In many rural areas, the hospital is the center of health care delivery. It is the central delivery point for emergency and acute care services and may also be the same for physician and long-term care services (Hartwell 1988). Yet despite the centrality of the rural hospital, many have been closing. Generally, over half of all hospital closures in any recent year has been in rural areas.

Rural hospitals have suffered from the greater levels of poverty in rural areas. Often residents lack insurance or the means to pay their hospital bills. Also, Medicaid and Medicare payment rates for rural hospitals are considerably less than for urban ones. Finally, many rural hospitals have found it increasingly difficult to compete with the expensive technology found in larger urban hospitals.

While there may soon be a physician surplus across the nation, rural areas continue to face a physician shortage. The physician-to-population ratio in small rural communities is 53 per 100,000 compared to 163 per 100,000 as the national average (Kindig et al. 1987).

There are several reasons why physicians may not care to practice in rural areas. First, the lack of hospital and other medical facilities may dissuade many physicians. Second, the lack of professional peers and consultation may discourage physicians' movement to rural areas. Third, the higher poverty rates of rural areas reduce the income potential of physicians. Fourth, rural areas' lack of cultural amenities may dissuade many physicians.

## DEVELOPMENT OF RURAL HMOs

Although it is more difficult to establish rural HMOs, they do have a long history. As early as the mid-1800s, industries such as logging and mining often had prepaid arrangements with physicians who would offer medical care to workers in isolated rural areas (Ross 1975). As noted in Chapter 2, the Elk City Cooperative grew out of the severe conditions of the depression and the need for low-cost health care in rural communities. The cooperative hired salaried physicians who provided health care to farmers who paid a fixed-sum payment. By the late 1930s, about 600,000 rural residents were members of prepaid plans similar to the Elk City model (Christianson 1989).

Many of the plans formed during the depression and World War II did not survive the intense opposition of local physicians. There was little further development of rural HMOs until the passage of the Health Maintenance Act of 1973. Sections of this act were expressly intended to encourage rural HMOs. Indeed, the Act required that at least 20 percent of the federal funds available for the development of HMOs be set aside for HMOs that attract two-thirds of their enrollees from rural areas.

Following an initial flurry of new rural HMOs after the passage of the 1973 HMO Act, the development of rural-based HMOs slowed (Christianson 1989). In fact, the "rural set aside funds" were never totally depleted during the seventies because of insufficient quality applications (Paley and Bickman 1979).

This slow development of rural HMOs reflects the numerous barriers to their development. First, the small and sparse population in rural areas makes it difficult for HMOs to acquire a sufficiently large membership. When an HMO has more members, it can spread capital and other fixed costs over more enrollees and thus reduce costs. Yet many HMOs in rural areas would have to attain 50 percent penetration of their local markets in order to achieve 10,000 members, which is a comparatively small HMO. Achieving 50 percent penetration of any market is not an easy task. In comparison, an HMO in a metropolitan area of one million could attain the same number of enrollees with only one percent of the market. Thus, the rural HMOs must appeal to a much broader cross-section of the population to achieve sufficient enrollment (Christianson and Shadle 1988).

Maintaining high enrollment levels in rural HMOs can be difficult because of the HMOs' high visibility in rural areas. If individuals are upset with the quality of their care in a rural HMO, they are likely to reach a larger proportion of the community than would be the case in urban areas. Such negative perceptions could produce a poor image that would be difficult for the HMO to overcome (Christianson et al. 1986).

Another barrier to the development of HMOs was the opposition of many rural physicians. Rural physicians who have practiced for some time in rural areas may often have had little contact with HMOs, and thus may have had misconceptions about the requirements for participation in an HMO. Moreover, doctors attracted to rural areas were more likely to value their independence and were often rugged individualists who were philosophically opposed to prepaid medicine.

Rural physicians often did not feel as much pressure as urban physicians for new patients. Given the lower physician-to-population ratio in rural areas, many rural physicians already had all of the patients they desired. Hence, they saw little incentive to join an HMO. Since a few physicians in a rural area often had nearly all the patients in the community, they sometimes had little reason to join an HMO. Since the HMO had limited capacity to increase the physicians' patient base, they had little incentive to accept the risk-sharing, the utilization reviews, and cost-containment strategies of the HMO as conditions for admission.

The lower level of income in many rural areas has meant that the real target population for an HMO is substantially less than the actual population (InterStudy, *Considerations in Developing a Rural HMO* 1988). If a large proportion of this lower-income population is without health insurance or benefits, and if many of these individuals are not covered by Medicaid, they cannot afford to participate in an HMO.

The type of industries and workforces in rural areas is not conducive to HMOs. Many urban HMOs generally appeal to large employers who provide extensive health benefits to a large number of employees. By concentrating on these large employers, urban HMOs can obtain large enrollments from a single narrowly focused marketing effort. This approach can maximize enrollment while minimizing marketing costs.

Most employers in rural areas are small and many may provide only minimal health care benefits. Also, many workers in rural areas are self-employed. Thus, rural HMOs must appeal to many more small employers. However, it is more difficult for an HMO to devise a plan that is attractive to many small employers rather than a few large ones. The HMO's marketing task becomes considerably more difficult and expensive.

Small employers often have fewer resources to spend on health care benefits. Hence, rural HMOs have a more difficult time providing cost-effective plans.

Agriculture is a major force in the economy of most rural areas. During the 1980s, this sector suffered major economic setbacks. As a result, rural HMOs often found a depressed and difficult economy in which to develop.

Another barrier to HMO growth in rural areas was the more general resistance to change often found in rural areas. Many rural residents were unfamiliar with the HMO concept and suspicious of HMOs' goals and operations. Therefore, a rural HMO's marketing task was further complicated by the general suspicions of the population.

Despite these barriers to rural HMO development, there was a resurgence of interest during the 1980s. There are several reasons for this renewed interest. First, as competition among HMOs in urban areas grew more intense, the urban HMOs looked to surrounding rural areas as viable areas for expansion. Thus, over one-third of all HMOs have some providers who practice in nonmetropolitan counties. Almost all of these HMOs are headquartered in urban counties.

While local physicians often opposed HMO development, more and more became fearful that neighboring urban HMOs would spread into their communities. Likewise, as roads and transportation improved in rural areas, and when rural residents could more easily travel to urban areas, rural doctors saw more and more patients opt for medical care in the city. Thus, rural physicians began to see rural HMOs as a response to the perceived competition from urban providers.

A large HMO may also move into a rural area in order to provide coverage for some of the employees of a large employer whose plant is located in an adjoining urban area. Similarly, as the number of for-profit HMOs increase, some may believe that they can realize a profit in rural areas (InterStudy, *Considerations in Developing a Rural HMO* 1988).

## FACTORS IN SUCCESSFUL RURAL HMOs

HMOs that have survived in rural areas have been particularly successful in obtaining community and provider support which in turn facilitated finding both adequate financing and sufficient enrollment. Of course, they also have managed to control costs. The success of rural HMOs have also rested on the appropriate type of organizational arrangements. These factors are discussed below.

### Obtaining Community Support

In most smaller communities, there is generally some resistance to change. A new HMO in a rural community symbolizes considerable change in the sensitive area of health care. The first and natural reaction of many residents will be suspicion. For some, prepaid HMOs may smack of ''socialized medicine,'' or government-sponsored medicine. Given this predisposition to suspicion, HMOs must make sizable efforts to obtain community support at the outset.

In smaller communities, there is much more informal and word-of-mouth contact. Rumors and complaints can quickly circulate across the area and undermine an HMO's marketing effort. Thus, HMOs must have community leaders and opinion makers involved in the HMO to counteract or influence the informal communication network.

During HMO development, town meetings may be called to educate and build support among the residents. Influential leaders may be asked to speak out in support of the HMO. Most rural federally qualified HMOs do not use the mandate against an employer. Such actions would antagonize the employer and could quickly lead to negative reactions throughout the community. Instead, the federal qualification is used as a symbol of the quality of the HMO (Christianson et al. 1986).

Rural HMOs have taken other measures to build community support. Many have affiliated with Blue Cross/Blue Shield in an effort to establish legitimacy in rural areas. Others have affiliated with clinics already established and respected in the community (Christianson et al. 1986).

It is particularly important that an urban-based HMO which is expanding into a rural area obtain the support of the community. It is very likely to be viewed as an outside stranger. Such HMOs should take great pains to educate and gain the acceptance of local community leaders (e.g., significant employers, civic leaders, ministers, and educators).

Successful HMOs select and use their boards of directors or advisory groups to develop community support. The initial directors should command respect across a broad section of the community. The selection of board members or advisory group members sends a clear message of what kind of organization the HMO will be (InterStudy, *Considerations in Developing a Rural HMO* 1988).

HMO administrators and heads of marketing should be selected who will have good relations with the community. While they need not be members of the local community, they should understand and have good rapport with rural residents. Prior residence in rural areas would be a definite plus.

### Acquiring Financing

Most new HMOs, particularly staff or group-model HMOs, need considerable capital to carry them through the initial years to a point of financially breaking even. This is a need of any new HMO, and it is particularly acute for rural HMOs (Christianson et al. 1986). Group practices are less common in rural areas and most are composed of only a few doctors who have limited resources to assist HMO development. Likewise, many rural hospitals are barely surviving. Thus, they are not in a position to subsidize the initial years of an HMO.

The type of HMO developed has considerable impact on the financing requirements. A staff-model HMO with salaried physicians and new facilities will demand much more capital than the expansion of an IPA model to physicians who already practice in a rural community.

The way most rural HMOs have obtained financing is from an established parent HMO in an urban area that is expanding into an adjoining rural area. Such HMOs bring administrative and financial structure as well as capital to the rural area.

### Obtaining the Support of Local Providers

Until very recently, most rural HMOs have been opposed by local doctors. As noted earlier, many rural physicians selected a rural practice because they valued their independence and were often philosophically opposed to HMOs. In addition, much physician opposition may have resulted from ignorance of HMOs combined with fear that they would undermine the physicians' income.

In rural areas, HMOs cannot afford the opposition of local physicians. Thus, new HMOs must pursue various strategies to reduce the opposition of physicians if not gain their cooperation. Perhaps the most successful strategy is to note that competition will bring HMOs to many rural areas, and it is best for physicians to be in a constructive leadership mode within an HMO rather than in a defensive, reactive position. Since many rural physicians now see urban-based HMOs to be potential competitors, they are more receptive to this approach (Christianson et al. 1986). Indeed, rural doctors recognize that with good highways and fast transportation, many of their former patients may refer themselves to physicians in urban areas.

Concern about urban competition is particularly useful in gaining physician cooperation in the development of a rural-based HMO as opposed to an urban-based HMO that is expanding into a rural area. The rural-based HMO can allow considerable authority to local physicians and can bring a distinctly rural perspective to plan management. On the other hand, urban-based HMOs expanding into rural areas have attempted to combine decentralized decision-making in the delivery of medical services with centralized administration of administrative activities such as marketing, claims processing and management information systems (Christianson et al. 1986).

Another strategy of reducing local physician opposition is to lessen concern about the HMO's impact on the physicians' income. Most rural HMOs attempt to refer patients within their service areas as much as possible. This tends to reduce physician concern that the HMO will move patients to the city. Some HMOs may choose to initially offer discounted fee-for-service compensation to rural doctors so to least interfere with their medical practices.

As rural HMOs need the support of local doctors, they also need the cooperation of local hospitals. Unlike urban areas, many rural communities have only one local hospital. Thus, the hospital may not be too interested in negotiating discounts or in risk-sharing with a new HMO. Moreover, rural hospitals tend to be in more difficult financial positions than urban hospitals. Hence, they are less likely to sponsor a rural-based HMO. In addition, since many rural hospitals have numerous empty beds, they may not welcome an HMO's attempts to decrease hospitalization.

Yet there are forces that encourage a rural hospital to cooperate with a rural HMO. Perceived competition or the threat of competition by urban hospitals is probably the main motivating factor. Like rural physicians, many rural hospitals recognize that more and more of their patients may choose to be hospitalized in larger, more sophisticated urban hospitals. Therefore, they may see an HMO as a way to control the potential loss of patients. New rural HMOs can capitalize on this fear.

The new HMO should stress its desire to utilize the local hospital and not send its patients to an adjoining urban facility. This is particularly important for an urban-based HMO that is expanding into a rural area. Such a decision may relieve some of the hospital's fears, and is probably more efficient since rural hospital costs are often significantly less than in urban areas.

### Selecting the Appropriate Organizational Structure

A rural HMO must decide several organization issues including the particular HMO type or model, whether to adopt a profit or not-for-profit status and whether to seek federal qualification status. When deciding upon an HMO model or type, most rural HMOs will not adopt a staff model. Most rural-based HMOs will not have sufficient capital to employ a staff of physicians when the new HMO is unsure of how many members it will enroll. The staff model, with its large salary and capital commitments, would be economically prohibitive for most rural-based HMOs.

It is possible that an urban-based HMO that is expanding into a rural area might employ the staff approach, particularly if it is already a staff-model HMO. However, importing a complete new staff of physicians into a rural area is certain to produce intense opposition from the local physicians who see an immediate threat to their practices. Thus, such an HMO could be in a very difficult situation with large fixed capital costs and intense local opposition.

The staff model might work in a rural area where there is a clear shortage of physicians. In such a situation, overworked rural doctors might accept outside providers. Yet even here, the HMO must make sure that the doctors recruited for the rural staff enjoy rural areas and will remain for some time in the area. Otherwise, there will be considerable turnover among the staff which will severely affect the HMO's reputation.

A group-model HMO is possible if there is a local group already practicing in the rural area that is willing to participate. Generally, such a group serves both fee-for-service and HMO members, and the physicians are reimbursed on a salaried basis (Christianson 1989).

Most rural HMOs are IPAs. This is because these are often the least expensive and least intrusive ways to introduce an HMO into a rural area. An urban-based HMO can expand into a rural community by contracting with the rural physicians practicing in the area. Comparatively little start-up costs are required. Likewise, if existing rural physicians decide to sponsor an HMO, it will probably be an IPA because it would least interfere with their practices.

Some rural HMOs using the IPA model have invited all local physicians to join the HMO. While this strategy reduces factionalism and promotes community acceptance of the plan, it may also bring physicians into the plan who do not practice a conservative style of medicine. HMOs who open their doors to all community physicians risk miscommunication about the basic goals and philosophy of the HMO. Physicians may believe that they have been misled. Thus, if all physicians are invited into an IPA, it probably should spend considerable time educating physicians about utilization control and review procedures (InterStudy, *Considerations in Developing a Rural HMO* 1988).

Most rural IPAs use discounted fee-for-service with a small "withhold" or risk-sharing arrangement. A few rural IPAs have used the "gatekeeper" approach where physicians are capitated for all or a major portion of the member's services. This approach allows an IPA to operate more like a group or staff model by placing the primary care physician in charge of care and dollars (InterStudy, *Considerations in Developing a Rural HMO* 1988). However, it is subject to problems as noted in Chapter 6.

In addition to selecting an appropriate model or type, rural HMOs must select either profit or not-for-profit status. During the seventies, nonprofit rural HMOs may have been encouraged by the availability of federal grants for some development costs. With the disappearance of federal money, nonprofit status may be less attractive. However, a nonprofit arrangement might arouse less suspicion in a rural community (InterStudy, *Considerations in Developing a Rural HMO* 1988). In any case, a nonprofit will not have to produce as much revenue per member in order for the plan to be financially stable.

On the other hand, for-profit status may provide better access to the capital needed to get the plan off the ground. Also, for-profit HMOs may be more attractive to providers if the financial plan indicates a profit. Moreover, some employers may believe that a for-profit HMO may be more professionally run and likely to be financially viable (InterStudy, *Considerations in Developing a Rural HMO* 1988).

A new rural HMO must also decide whether to seek federal qualification. Federal qualification could either enhance or impede an HMO's reputation in a rural community. If there are concerns about "socialized medicine," federal qualification may appear as more government intrusion. On the other hand, federal qualification could be viewed as a sign of quality.

Federal qualification requires considerable reporting requirements. While large urban HMOs may have staff who process such documents, a small rural-based HMO may not have sufficient staff to easily meet the reporting requirements (InterStudy, *Considerations in Developing a Rural HMO* 1988).

There may be other reasons that smaller rural-based HMOs may have second thoughts about federal qualification. Such status requires an HMO to offer a comprehensive set of benefits. These may be too expensive for a small HMO and/or place it at a competitive disadvantage with traditional insurance plans. The federal status restricts an HMO's ability to fashion particular benefits for a particular employer or customer. Likewise, federal restrictions on copayments and deductibles may restrict an HMO's cost-containment efforts and its ability to generate revenue. Moreover, community rating, as required by the federal requirements, may produce HMO rates that are not competitive.

On the other hand, if a rural HMO intends to enroll the Medicare population in the community, federal status is a reasonable objective. Since the percentage of elderly residents in many rural communities tends to be higher, many rural HMOs will seek to enroll them and should probably seek federal status.

### Obtaining Sufficient Enrollment

During the early 1970s, it was believed that successful rural HMOs needed 20,000 to 30,000 members to be financially viable (Christianson and Shadle 1988). While rural HMOs have survived with much lower numbers, obtaining sufficient enrollment remains a problem in many rural areas.

In sparsely populated regions, successful HMOs must attain a much larger market population than the typical urban HMOs must achieve. This is made more difficult by the general lack of large employers who could provide large percentages of an HMO's total enrollment. Moreover, many of the smaller employers may not provide health care benefits. In addition, many in rural areas are self-employed and thus must purchase their own health insurance.

As a result of these differences, many rural HMOs must attract more individuals who pay their own premiums. Since HMO premiums tend to be higher than those for insurance plans which generally provide fewer benefits, the less healthy, who believe that they will need the HMO's comprehensive benefits, may be the most willing to pay the higher premiums. Thus, rural HMOs are more concerned about adverse selection. Of course, if a disproportionate number of the enrollees are ill, the premiums will continue upward thereby driving away the healthy who are looking for lower premiums and fewer benefits. In order to prevent such adverse selection, some rural HMOs use medical screening tests for potential enrollees to determine who will be accepted.

Since rural HMOs contract with many smaller employers and with individuals, they must custom fashion many plans and packages for these smaller buyers. This need to fashion a particular plan for small employers or individual buyers may limit rural HMOs' desire for federal qualification. Federal status requires an HMO to offer a full range of benefits that costs more than the small buyer's ability to pay. Moreover, the community ratings often used by federal HMOs produce premiums that are not competitive. Hence, some rural HMOs may forgo federal qualification in order to maintain flexibility in benefit packages and to be competitive in price.

### Containing Costs

While rural HMOs historically have not faced as much competition from other HMOs as do those HMOs in urban areas, they nevertheless have several reasons to closely monitor costs. First, rural residents often have lower incomes and find it more difficult to pay premiums. Thus, they are more price sensitive. This is particularly significant since a larger percentage of rural HMOs' enrollments is composed of individually purchased membership. Likewise, the smaller employers in rural areas are often less able to pay larger premiums.

Second, rural HMOs face tough competition from traditional insurance plans that offer fewer benefits combined with higher deductibles and copayments. This combination can result in significantly lower premiums that appeal to price sensitive buyers. Conversely, rural HMOs often have more comprehensive benefits with limited, if any, deductibles and copayments. This is particularly true for federally qualified HMOs. As a result, rural HMOs have to be very concerned about controlling costs in order to compete with traditional insurance plans.

Third, rural HMOs in recent years have faced ever-increasing competition from urban HMOs that are seeking to expand into adjoining rural areas.

Rural HMOs, like urban HMOs, use financial risk-sharing by providers, utilization review, and prior authorization for hospital admissions and specialists to control costs. In addition, rural HMOs have borrowed staff and management systems from sponsoring organizations. For example, a business manager for a sponsoring physician group might serve as a part-time HMO administrator (Christianson and Shadle 1988). Similarly, rural HMOs have contracted out some activities such as maintenance of enrollee data systems to larger organizations.

Most rural physicians have been willing to accept financial risk-sharing because of the increased competition from urban-based providers. Likewise, rural hospitals have been willing to share more risk; however, the precarious financial plight of many rural hospitals restricts their capacity to do so. Thus, while rural HMOs hold out the opportunity to reduce the flight of rural patients to urban hospitals, they could plunge an already tottering hospital into financial collapse through aggressive risk-sharing. Of course, such an outcome is not in the HMO's interest when there is only one rural hospital and when the urban alternative is very likely to have significantly higher rates. Therefore, rural HMOs must be more concerned than urban HMOs about the financial impact of their negotiated risk-sharing on the rural hospitals.

Although rural HMOs use some pre-admission review and concurrent review, most rely more heavily on education of physicians and feedback about practice patterns as the primary way to control utilization. Rural HMOs do not use pre-admission certification requirements as much as do urban HMOs (Christianson et al. 1986).

## RURAL-BASED VERSUS URBAN-BASED HMOs IN RURAL AREAS

Two kinds of HMOs serve rural areas—rural-based and urban-based HMOs. Approximately one-third of all HMOs in 1984 served rural areas (Christianson 1989). However, the vast majority of these HMOs were urban-based HMOs which expanded into adjoining rural areas. Only a handful were rural-based HMOs. There are a number of benefits and problems associated with each type.

Rural-based HMOs may be more economical in that rural physicians often practice a more conservative style of medicine and charge lower rates. Also, a rural-based HMO would not be subsidizing urban subscribers in the same HMO whose costs are likely to be higher.

Rural-based HMOs also provide an opportunity to reduce the relative isolation of rural physicians. For example, the doctors could interact and share information through participation in utilization review and quality assurance procedures (Christianson and Shadle 1988).

Rural-based HMOs also permit local control over medical decisions. Urban decision criteria and protocols may not always be appropriate in rural settings. This may be particularly true as regards hospital admissions and discharges. Rural patients may be admitted more readily into hospitals because of the lack of free-standing clinics, home health care services, and other alternatives to hospitalization. Also, the lower costs for hospital stays in rural areas may result in hospitalization being more economically competitive with other forms of treatment.

Rural-based HMOs may take greater care to maintain existing rural-based medical care (physicians and hospitals). Urban-based HMOs might be more inclined to bring rural patients to urban areas for care.

Along with these potential benefits, rural-based HMOs also have potential problems. Rural-based HMOs could experience relatively large per-member start-up costs because of the need to spread fixed costs over a small membership. These higher costs could jeopardize the financial stability of the rural-based HMO. Of course, the insolvency and failure of a rural-based HMO could do great harm to already fragile rural care systems.

Another disadvantage of rural-based HMOs is that they may be unlikely to profit from the advanced technology and expertise found in urban medical centers. If rural-based HMOs limit referrals to urban specialists and hospitals because of the financial interest of the rural-based HMO, then this unfortunate outcome is even more likely to occur.

On the other hand, urban-based HMOs have certain potential advantages. Because of their larger enrollments, they are able to spread administrative costs over a larger group and thus attain lower per-member administrative costs. Similarly, it may be less expensive for an existing urban-based HMO to spread into an adjoining rural area than it would be to start a completely new HMO in the same area. Much of the administrative structure would already be in place.

Urban-based HMOs may also have more sophisticated and advanced utilization review procedures. In addition, their larger data bases may allow them to better evaluate physicians' practice patterns (Christianson and Shadle 1988). Furthermore, since the urban-based HMO is less dependent upon local physicians, they may be more effective in implementing utilization and cost-control procedures. Finally, urban-based HMOs may be best able to develop linkages between rural physicians and urban specialists and between rural hospitals and larger tertiary care institutions in urban centers.

Along with these potential advantages, urban-based HMOs suffer certain potential risks. While urban-based HMOs have lower per-member administrative costs, their medical costs per member may be higher because of the higher medical costs of their urban members. Thus, if premiums for rural enrollees are established on the actual experience of all HMO enrollees both rural and urban, the rural members may be subsidizing the higher medical costs of their fellow urban members.

In some large urban-based HMOs, there is a danger that the rural component of the HMO's membership is so small that it fails to get much attention and adequate resources from the HMO. Similarly, if an urban-based HMO cannot reach its profit targets in a rural area, it may abruptly terminate its contracts. Of course, this could have a very detrimental impact on an already fragile local medical network.

On the other hand, if the urban-based HMO is meeting its profit targets, it may gradually increase the use of urban specialists and medical centers, particularly if the HMO is sponsored by physicians and hospitals in the urban area.

After a substantial portion of a rural population is enrolled in an urban-based HMO, the rural physicians may have no alternative but to accept the HMO's gradual policy of referring more and more patients to urban specialists and hospitals. Of course, such a policy would tend to undermine the local medical infrastructure.

## CONCLUSION

HMOs in rural areas have been growing rapidly in recent years. Most of this expansion has resulted from the expansion of urban-based HMOs into rural areas. Thus, rural physicians and hospitals often do not have a choice of whether there is to be an HMO in their community. The more likely choice or decision is whether rural providers will form their own HMO or join an urban-based one. Likewise, rural providers may increasingly see their active participation in an HMO as one of few viable ways to reduce the continual erosion of their practices by the self-referral of their patients to specialists and providers in urban areas. Thus, rural physicians and hospitals appear much more willing to accept both the financial risk-sharing and utilization review implicit in HMOs. Therefore, it appears likely that HMO growth in rural areas will continue.

# 9

# HMOs and Preferred Provider Organizations

Preferred provider organizations (PPOs) are the chief competitors to HMOs in managed care markets. In recent years, they have been expanding at phenomenal rates. In theory, they appear to offer real advantages for all concerned—consumers, purchasers and providers.

## DEFINITION AND CHARACTERISTICS OF PPOs

Because of the great variety of PPOs and their continuing evolution, it is difficult to provide a precise definition of them. However, there are certain commonalities often present in most PPOs including:

a. formal contractual arrangements,
b. a select panel of providers,
c. an emphasis on cost efficiency,
d. marketing to purchasers as opposed to users,
e. some flexibility in choice of providers together with financial incentives to use selected providers.

A formal contractual structure is present in most PPOs (Barger et al. 1985). The PPO is a legal entity which initiates contracts with several groups including purchasers of health care such as employers, and providers of health care such as physicians, hospitals, pharmacies, nursing homes, etc. Even a small PPO typically contracts with more than 500 physicians and 15 hospitals. A larger PPO may contract with over 3,000 doctors and several hundred hospitals.

PPOs also include a select panel of providers. In theory, most PPOs hope that their panels contain the most cost efficient providers who provide the highest quality care. However, practice falls somewhat short of theory. PPOs' first goal may be to build a network of providers that can cover a market or geographical region. Thus, PPOs may first be more concerned about having sufficient providers rather than efficient ones. Yet, if PPOs fail to establish controls over entry, they will eventually run into marketing and financial problems. Therefore, most PPOs will develop screening criteria to determine who is admitted to the panel and who can remain.

Since PPOs' chief goal is to provide more cost efficient health care, all must emphasize cost containment in order to survive. There are several ways that a PPO can control costs including (1) obtaining discounts from providers, (2) using payment schemes that transfer some risk to the providers, and (3) using utilization controls.

PPOs generally sell their product directly to major purchasers. Early PPOs directed their marketing efforts directly at corporations that self-funded their insurance and to labor-union trusts (Barger et al. 1985). Subsequently, PPOs sought to sell their services to third party administrators, employee benefits brokers and insurance companies.

Unlike many HMOs, most PPOs allow subscribers to use providers outside of its panel. However, if the PPO is to be successful and if it is to live up to its marketing promises, it must channel its subscribers to its selected providers. Therefore, PPOs provide rewards to subscribers who use its doctors and hospitals. For example, an employee who normally pays a $200 deductible and a 20 percent copayment may not have to pay any deductible or copayment when using a PPO provider. Or a broader range of services may be available from the PPO panel of providers.

In theory, PPOs provide benefits to purchasers of health care as well as providers and consumers. Purchasers' primary desire is for cost savings. These may be achieved through discounts. However, discounts alone may not represent true savings. Thus, purchasers also look for cost containment through utilization review as well as other innovative payment mechanisms such as per diem payments which involve some form of risk sharing.

Generally, providers form or join PPOs in order to maintain or expand market shares and patient volume. A poll of hospitals involved in PPOs revealed that 95 percent did so to increase market share or increase occupancy rates (Perspectives 1983).

Providers also like the rapid payment provided by most PPOs. Outside of PPOs, payments to physicians may often take 40 days to complete. For hospitals, payments may not be completed for 60 days. In PPOs, payments are often made within 7 to 10 days. This promptness improves cash flow for providers and allows providers greater return on their earnings. PPOs also avoid the 5 to 10 percent bad debt problems that providers often encounter when trying to collect.

Most PPOs maintain the fee-for-service reimbursement system which providers find attractive. Providers prefer fee-for-service in that it does not place providers at risk.

Consumers like PPOs because they often can forego deductibles and copayments when the preferred panel of providers is used. Consumers may also benefit from the utilization and quality reviews found in PPOs. Consumers also like the ability to use non-PPO providers whenever they wish, providing they pay deductibles and copayments.

## GROWTH AND DEVELOPMENT OF PPOs

During the 1980s, the numbers of PPOs increased dramatically as did the number of employees in plans with a PPO option. In 1981, fewer than 110 PPOs were operational (Barger et al. 1985). By 1985, almost 300 PPOs were available in the United States, and approximately 6 million employees had a PPO option (Rice et al. 1985). By 1989, some 18.3 million workers were covered by almost 700 operational PPOs. Based on these figures, over 42 million Americans (including dependents) are eligible to use PPOs, given an average family size of 2.3 people (Marion 1989).

There are several reasons for such rapid growth. The rapid health care cost increases of the late 1970s and early 1980s convinced employers that they had to find ways to combat such increases. At the same time, the number of physicians was increasing dramatically as was the number of empty hospital beds. These conditions favored the rapid development of HMOs. Since health care providers generally find PPOs much more acceptable than HMOs, the success of HMOs paradoxically contributed to the rapid rise of PPOs. Providers who sought a managed care arrangement to compete with the HMOs turned to the PPOs. PPOs preserved the fee-for-service payments and represented less intrusion into practice and payment practices than did HMOs.

It should be noted that the number of employees covered by PPOs may be inflated. Many employers provide several PPO options to their employees. Therefore, some PPOs may be reporting the same employees or doublecounting the same individuals. Moreover, the number of employees who actually use the PPO option may be much less than the number covered by the PPO. In addition, some may use the option for some but not all medical care.

PPOs are owned and sponsored by different groups. Providers such as hospitals and doctors are major owners (28 percent of PPOs) as are insurance companies (33 percent). Indeed, insurance companies own seven of the top ten PPOs in the country with a combined enrollment of approximately three million employees. Some companies that self-fund health care for their employees also sponsor PPOs.

Corporate PPO chains are those that operate PPOs in more than one state. The 33 national chains have over 448 PPOs that cover nearly twelve million workers or 65 percent of all employees covered (Marion 1989).

PPOs tend to be concentrated in the larger states. California has 149 plans with over six million covered workers. Other states with large numbers of covered employees include Colorado, Minnesota, Alabama, Georgia, Tennessee, Ohio, and Pennsylvania. PPOs tend to have the highest market penetration in the West, especially California, and the lowest in the East.

## COST CONTROLS IN PPOs

At the start of the PPO movement, discounts were the primary tool in PPOs' attempts to provide less expensive health care. Over time, more and more PPOs have turned to other methods to reduce costs, including selecting more efficient providers, implementing utilization review, and requiring more risk-sharing by providers.

### Discounts

Today, approximately one-third of all doctors under contract with PPOs are paid with discounted fees. The average discount is 22 percent from usual customary and reasonable (UCR) charges (Marion 1989). Nearly half of all hospitals contracting with PPOs use discounts from UCR charges. Hospital discounts average about 15 percent (Foster Higgins 1988). However, discounts do not discourage the more pernicious impacts of the fee-for-service system. In fact, with discounted fee-for-service, doctors may be encouraged to deliver more health care in order to recoup money lost through discounts. In one of the few empirical studies on this question, Garnick et al. (1990) found this to be apparently the case.

Discounts could actually increase total health care costs if the number of services increases following the use of discounts or if the discounted fees are actually higher than the fees usually charged by a physician. For example, if the PPO discount is 90 percent of the UCR charges in a region, but the doctors under contract with the PPO historically charged only 85 percent of the region's UCR charges, then the discounted fees could actually be more expensive than those the doctors would have charged without any contract with the PPO. Moreover, if the doctors most inclined to seek a contract with a PPO are those who most need or want additional patients, then they already could be offering fees below the region's average UCR charges. Thus, paradoxically, the discounted fees could be more than the doctors' usual fees.

A similar phenomenon could occur with discounts by hospitals. Hospitals could deliver more services, and thus drive up the total costs even while providing discounts. As a result of these concerns, PPOs have moved to use other methods, such as selecting more efficient providers, to control costs.

### Selecting Efficient Providers

PPOs must select efficient providers and channel their enrollees to these providers if PPOs are to realize true savings. This necessity is at the core of the PPO concept. Otherwise, PPOs could actually encourage cost increases by sending consumers to the less efficient providers who, even with discounts, are providing more expensive, less efficient services. Indeed, employers primarily join PPOs for their assumed ability to channel employees to cost-efficient providers. This channeling effect was noted by nearly half of all employers as the primary reason for using the PPO while only 15 percent mentioned discounts (Billet and Cantor 1985).

Selecting efficient physicians involves determining who (1) offers quality health services, (2) has hospital practice patterns that result in below average stays and total charges per patient, and (3) uses inpatient resources sparingly (Barger et al. 1985). However, these are often difficult to accomplish. Data on quality and practice patterns are rarely available and are often subjective. Yet, even when data on charges and lengths of stay are available, one may not know the third component, that is, unnecessary hospitalization. Indeed, if a physician hospitalizes those that truly do not require it, the physician could have lower inpatient stays and total charges because nonacute patients were admitted.

Because efficiency data is difficult to obtain, many PPOs do not seek it. Moreover, since a PPO could contract with over a thousand doctors, obtaining claims data on each one would be very difficult indeed. Thus, it is not surprising that surveys have revealed none of the top ten PPOs in the country was selective in contracting with physicians, and only 23 percent of the other PPOs were deemed selective (Gabel et al. 1986). PPOs often look at other selection criteria such as membership in medical societies, admission to the medical staff of selected hospitals, malpractice record, and board certification. Less than 20 percent of PPOs actually analyze claims data of doctors prior to their acceptance into the PPO (Gabel et al. 1986).

Once admitted into a PPO, stringent efficiency criteria may be used to guide practice patterns, but they are not generally used as a prerequisite for entry. However, more PPOs are attempting to better screen physicians prior to entry. For example, some PPOs ask the hospital with which they wish to contract to provide data on patient days within Diagnostically Related Groups (DRGs) for each doctor on staff. In this way, patient days above average and charges above average can be computed. Of course, the PPO would then attempt to contract with doctors who have average or below average stays and costs.

Another system for measuring efficiency is the Non-Acute Profile in which a sample of patient charts are reviewed to see if specific acute conditions or acute care services were noted on the charts for a particular day. Then the number of non-acute days among the sampled charts are computed. Such analysis within diagnostically-related groups across different physicians can reveal which doctors seem to have a higher number of non-acute days in the sample. Such physicians may be admitting too early, discharging too late, or admitting non-acute cases. In any event, they may not be the efficient doctors with whom PPOs wish to contract.

If PPOs are primarily interested in expanding their network of providers as quickly as possible in order to provide ample and easy access to medical care, they may be less concerned, at least at the start of a PPO, in selecting the most cost-efficient physicians. Also, if a PPO attempts to keep out the less efficient, it could antagonize many physicians. In any case, whatever admission criteria PPOs adopt, they must be uniform from doctor to doctor in order to avoid any potential legal risk.

PPOs must also use care in selecting cost-efficient hospitals. Determining the efficiency of hospitals, however, is also complex. If PPOs have been established by a hospital or group of hospitals, they are not interested in determining their own efficiency for purposes of deciding which hospitals to use. Indeed, they established the PPO to use their own facilities.

Even PPOs sponsored by groups other than hospitals will have a difficult time determining hospital efficiency. Perhaps this is why fewer than one-third of PPOs actually analyze hospital costs when selecting hospitals (Gabel et al. 1986). Indeed, about 60 percent of HMOs used location as the prime consideration in selecting hospitals. Also, PPOs may be just as concerned about service mix when selecting a hospital as they are about costs. Moreover, they may be uninterested in efficiency if the hospital offers large discounts from average charges, or if the hospital is willing to engage in risk-sharing arrangements with the PPO. Of course, if there are major inefficiencies in a hospital which offers discounts, then it is safe to assume that the hospital is passing along the costs of the discounts to other purchasers who have less influence and less ability to negotiate discounts.

For PPOs that wish to investigate efficiency, important data must be collected. The basic data is average cost per day or per admission. There can, however, be much variance in these data even within the same community. Such data can be influenced by several factors such as the case mix of patients. The severity level of patients can dramatically affect these figures (Barger et al. 1985). Yet, there are crude measures by which to assess costs per case when one controls for or holds constant the hospital's case mix. In other words, one can take the case mix of a hospital over a particular period of time and predict, using national averages for particular cases, what the hospital's costs should be. If the hospital's costs are high, then the hospital may be less efficient than a hospital with lower than predicted costs.

### Utilization Review in PPOs

As a result of not being able to always select the most efficient providers, PPOs implement utilization review to control costs. Preadmission certification and concurrent review are used by nearly all PPOs. Mandatory second opinions for surgery and retrospective reviews are also used extensively.

### Risk-Sharing Arrangements

Most doctors in PPOs do not share much of the risk in treating patients. Almost two-thirds are paid according to a fee schedule, and another third is paid with discounted fees. Thus, the doctors are paid an agreed sum for every service delivered. At this time, relatively few doctors in PPOs are paid by capitation, which would involve considerably more risk-sharing. Likewise, relatively few participate in risk-sharing pools which are funded by withholds from fees.

In comparison, many more hospitals engage in a form of risk-sharing. While 47 percent of hospitals contracting with PPOs in 1988 had payments based on discounted charges, 35 percent were paid per-diem rates. Another 10 percent were paid using diagnostically related groups (DRGs), and 5 percent received usual and customary charges (Marion 1989). The largest PPOs most often used per diem and DRG-based prices exclusively in contracts with hospitals.

Per diem payments represent risk-sharing by hospitals. Unlike billed charges, per diem payments are all-inclusive payments that offer incentives for efficient daily hospital performance. The hospital as well as the purchaser assumes some of the financial risk for treating each patient. However, it should be noted that hospitals are not penalized for excessive lengths of stay. They are reimbursed. Thus, it is not in a hospital's financial interest to keep stays at a minimum.

It is in the hospital's interest to keep expenditures per day to a minimum under per diem payments. However, hospitals may have relatively little control over such expenditures since physicians order most of the ancillary services that contribute to costs. Of course, the hospitals that are most likely to benefit from per-diem payments are those with efficient medical staff.

With per-diem reimbursement, the purchaser can cap the payment made per day and thus is able to make reasonable projections concerning total hospital costs. The risk is that lengths of stay will be longer than anticipated. Thus, PPOs must rely on effective utilization review, particularly concurrent review, to reduce or prevent unnecessarily lengthy stays.

Hospitals encounter risk under per diem payments when there is a case-mix imbalance. The daily cost of paying for a person in intensive care is much greater than the cost of routine pediatric surgical care, for example. Therefore, a hospital will incur a substantial loss if it receives per diem payments and has a larger than expected number of burn cases, heart surgeries, or other critical cases. For this reason, some hospitals and PPOs negotiate per-diem payments and lengths of stay based on DRGs.

Some PPOs negotiate payments based on admission. In other words, the hospital receives a set payment per admission that does not vary with the length of stay. Most such payments are based on differential payments for admissions in different DRGs. This type of hospital payment forces the hospital to consider the fundamental underlying problem of hospital inefficiency, that is, physician practice patterns (Barger et al. 1985). Hospitals under such a payment scheme cannot afford doctors with inefficient styles of practice.

If PPOs and hospitals wish to place physicians more at risk for health care services, several plans could be pursued. For example, the hospital could contract either on a per diem or per admission basis with the PPO. As an incentive for doctors, the hospital could agree to divide any surplus from PPO payments over costs with the physicians. Of course, the anticipated or contracted costs for each admission versus the real cost would have to be computed for each doctor in order to decide which doctors would share in the surplus and to what extent. Moreover, the hospital would face a political problem in deciding how to deal with physicians who consistently prescribed services that were more costly than the PPO payment.

Another possible method of risk-sharing is for the PPO to allocate to each physician's account a predetermined amount for each patient hospitalized. This amount could be based on per diem or per admission payments. In addition, it could be DRG specific. The essence of such a plan is that each individual doctor becomes responsible for payments to the hospital.

Thus, when a doctor's patient has a less expensive or less lengthy stay in a hospital than what was predicted and contracted for, the doctor would reap the benefits. Conversely, if the stay was longer and/or more expensive, the doctor would share the risk. Under such a plan, the PPO might not contract with any hospital. Contracts would be entered only with physicians who would be free to use any facility they wished.

### Channeling Consumers to PPO Providers

If PPOs are to operate as planned, they should direct consumers to less costly PPO-selected providers. PPOs rely upon both incentives and disincentives in trying to achieve this outcome. About three-fourths of PPOs offer lower deductibles as incentives to use PPO providers (Rice et al. 1985). However, deductibles are not eliminated in PPOs; rather they are lower (over $150) than they would be if non-preferred providers were used (Rice et al. 1989).

Often the coinsurance rate in conventional insurance plans is 20 percent. Likewise, for workers in PPOs the coinsurance rate is usually 20 percent when they use nonpreferred providers. When they use the PPO providers, the coinsurance is much more likely to be in the 0 to 10 percent range (Rice et al. 1989).

When marketing PPO plans to their employees, employers face a dilemma. If they wish to encourage employees to use the PPO providers because they offer discounts and/or because they are more efficient providers, they may offer low or no deductibles and coinsurance. Yet, offering "free" care to employees might subvert the PPO's cost-containment efforts by encouraging greater consumer demand for the "free" services (Rice et al. 1989). Therefore, employers apparently have decided to require a significant annual deductible of all individuals (both in and out of PPO plans) in order to control insurance-induced demand, but to provide low coinsurance rates to attract employees to PPOs' providers (Rice et al. 1989).

PPOs can also encourage greater use of preferred providers by providing additional health benefits such as well-baby care and physicals to those who use the PPO option. Approximately 25 percent of all PPOs provide additional health benefits to employees when they use preferred hospitals and doctors (Gabel et al. 1986).

The effectiveness of PPOs' channeling efforts is often unclear. Indeed, fewer than one in four PPOs are able to estimate the extent that subscribers actually use the preferred providers (Gabel et al. 1986). Another study revealed that only 1 in 18 physicians who contracted with a PPO had actually seen any PPO patients (Johns et al. 1985). Obviously, if a PPO is able to reduce costs dramatically, but can attract only a small percentage of a firm's employees to selected providers, it will not be able to realize significant savings.

### PPOs and Savings in Health Care Costs

The ability of PPOs to realize real cost savings for employers depends on (1) their ability to offer more efficient preferred providers, (2) their ability to channel employees to these providers, and (3) which employees (sick or healthy) use the PPO providers for which services (most expensive or least expensive).

As we have already seen, it is not clear that PPOs make strong efforts to recruit the most efficient providers. However, most PPOs do make vigorous efforts to promote efficient service through extensive utilization reviews. Similarly, about half of PPOs have taken steps to add physician profiling as part of their utilization review system, and many more are considering such systems (de Lissovoy et al. 1987). With physician profiling, PPOs collate all expenditures relating to an enrollee's episode of care and assign these charges to a responsible physician. Over time, it is possible to compare a particular physician's pattern of expenditures with his or her peers and to identify outliers. Of course, this analysis is useful only if PPOs are prepared to terminate the contracts of those physicians who will not modify their practice patterns. Surveys indicate that more than one-third of PPOs have terminated physician contracts as a result of noncompliance with utilization review or for other reasons (de Lissovoy et al. 1987). Apparently PPOs are more and more prepared to release physicians.

In addition to having efficient providers, PPOs must channel patients to such providers if they are to be cost-effective. While PPOs use a variety of incentives described earlier to accomplish this end, there is comparatively little research on how effective PPOs are in doing this. Research in one PPO by Diehr and others (1987) indicated that 50 percent of those eligible used the preferred provider in any given year, but it was unknown if and where the others obtained medical care and how they paid for it.

The Rand Corporation is examining the experience of six large employers that offer a PPO option in their employee benefit plans. Preliminary results from three firms in this study show that employees select PPO providers at widely varying rates. Over 60 percent of employees in one firm used the PPO, while only 37 percent and 13 percent of the employees in the other two firms used PPO providers (Ginsburg et al. 1987).

Another study of patient choice of providers by Wouters and Hester (1988) indicated that 32 percent of the employees used PPO providers. Similarly, approximately 30 percent of the employees used the PPO ambulatory services; however, only 12 percent used the PPO hospital.

This limited research suggests that employee use of PPO providers can vary widely, and use often depends on (1) the differentials in premiums and cost-sharing among the available options, (2) prior use of and satisfaction with medical providers, and (3) accessibility of the preferred medical providers and facilities.

Of course, the type of employee who selects the PPO option can also affect the PPO's ability to realize cost savings. In other words, if primarily healthy employees select the PPO, its true capacity to reduce costs is less than its apparent capacity. This is the same issue of biased selection that we reviewed in reference to HMO membership in Chapter 3.

While considerable research on biased selection has been done on membership in HMOs, little has been completed on biased selection in PPOs. It is more difficult to define membership in a PPO than membership in an HMO. Though some PPOs have formal enrollments similar to HMO enrollments, many do not. In any case, such enrollment would not define PPOs' effective membership since one of the key elements of a PPO is the freedom to select a non-PPO provider on a service-by-service basis.

In a typical PPO, the decision to use a PPO provider is made at the time service is needed, not at the time of enrollment. The individual's choice of provider is a balancing of the advantages of being able to reduce costs by use of a PPO provider versus the disadvantages of having to change preexisting physician relationships (Hester et al. 1987). The attractiveness of economic savings depends on the individual's income, out-of-pocket costs, time costs and the transition costs of switching providers. While those who are poor health risks might be the most attracted by the PPOs' lower costs, they are also the most likely to have established provider ties that they are least willing to break.

PPO membership is best defined operationally by including those individuals who actually use the PPO for service (Hester et al. 1987). Yet there can be various levels of "use" in any particular period of time. For example, if someone used a PPO physician for six routine visits during a year but used a non-PPO hospital for a major operation during the same time, is this person a PPO member?

Some research has classified membership according to the percent of an individual's total health care charges that are allocated to PPO providers (Hester et al. 1987). Using this definition, strong PPO users (those with over 50 percent of all charges in a PPO) tended to be younger employees who were hired more recently. No significant differences were found in education level, marital status and family size (Hester et al. 1987). Also, the strong PPO users' health care expenditures prior to using the PPO option was only 50 percent that of the non-PPO users. Similarly, health status surveys revealed the PPO users were a significantly healthier group than the weak or non-PPO users (Hester et al. 1987).

The same research revealed that the weak PPO users were a very ill population that required large amounts of health care services but used the PPO for only small amounts of minor services. They were willing to experiment with a new provider for less serious problems, and the financial incentives carried more weight in such cases (Hester et al. 1987).

Diehr et al. (1987) found that those who used a PPO only tended to be healthier than those who used both PPO and non-PPO providers. Those who did not use PPO providers exclusively tended to have greater incidence of cancer and hypertension.

Ginsburg et al. (1987) found that PPO participants tended to be younger and presumably healthier employees. However, when responses to health status questionnaires were compared, there were no consistent differences between PPO and non-PPO participants. On the other hand, PPO participants were less likely to have chronic health conditions such as hypertension. This research is preliminary, but it does tend to indicate that PPO users may be younger and have less chronic preexisting health conditions.

Although little empirical research exists on selection bias into PPOs, that which does exist indicates that those who are younger and who have fewer ties to medical care providers, and thus who are apparently healthier are more likely to use PPOs. Those with extensive medical care ties to non-PPO providers are least likely to use PPO providers, and if they do use them, it is for comparatively minor problems.

Most research which explores costs for PPO and non-PPO users in the same firm indicates that costs for PPO users are from 6 percent to 66 percent less than costs for non-PPO users (Barger et al. 1985, Leal 1987, Hester et al. 1987, and Diehr et al. 1988). Of course, these differentials could simply be the result of lower utilization by the PPO users. Indeed, this appears to be the case in several studies (Hester et al. 1987, Diehr et al. 1988). Since we know that the limited research available indicates favorable selection into PPOs, some of the savings may result from such selection rather than more efficient provision of medical services by PPO providers.

However, employers believe that PPOs do reduce their total costs. Billett and Cantor (1985) found that nearly half of the employers in their survey believe PPOs reduced total medical care costs. Likewise, a 1988 national survey of employers found that 60 percent of the respondents believed their PPOs were effective in controlling their health care costs. However, most of these employers probably did not know if there was biased favorable selection in their PPOs.

## ANTITRUST CONCERNS ABOUT PPOs

One of the chief legal issues facing PPOs involves antitrust implications. Since a PPO by its very nature is some combination of providers who were and are competitors, it could limit competition and violate the Sherman Antitrust Act. Indeed, the Supreme Court in 1982 ruled in *Arizona v. Maricopa County Medical Society* that agreements among physicians to establish maximum fee schedules constituted price fixing and thus were violations of federal antitrust statutes.

The Maricopa decision emphasizes the importance of sponsorship of a PPO when examining whether the PPO represents an unreasonable restraint of trade. A PPO sponsored by providers must be more careful to avoid violating antitrust law than a PPO sponsored by a third party, an employer, or an insurer. What may appear very appropriate and pro-competitive for one sponsor may look much more suspicious when done by providers who are supposedly competitors.

Providers who wish to form a PPO should probably consider a joint venture that includes a separate PPO entity in which they pool capital and share ownership and risk. The separate entity negotiates fees and contracts with individual providers and contracts for administrative services. However, sponsorship of a joint venture model PPO might also be illegal if much of a local market were influenced by the PPO. The intent of the sponsors, and the PPO's effect on competition would be critical in deciding the case.

Antitrust laws also prohibit group boycotts or refusals to deal. Providers who are excluded from PPO membership could charge that their ability to trade has been damaged by a PPO. However, if a provider who is excluded from a PPO is able to compete with the PPO by joining or organizing another PPO or by individually competing with the PPO, then it is difficult to show refusal to deal. This is particularly true when the PPO's intent is clearly not to restrain trade, and when the criteria for membership in the PPO are reasonable and consistently applied.

Providers and purchasers who enter into a PPO agreement could be accused of an exclusive dealing arrangement and thus be in violation of antitrust law (Barger et al. 1985). However, the purchaser does not determine from whom PPO enrollees will seek care; rather the enrollee makes the choice of PPO or non-PPO provider. Thus, there is no antitrust violation even when the purchase provides an incentive to use the preferred providers. Antitrust laws do not prevent the encouragement of economically rational behavior.

In general, antitrust law has not been a serious obstacle to PPO development. If the intent of the sponsors is to provide the best possible price for services and not to impede the ability of any provider to compete on the basis of price, the PPO will probably not violate antitrust law (Barger et al. 1985).

## COMPARISON OF HMOs AND PPOs

HMOs and PPOs can be compared along a number of dimensions. However, as someone has noted, "If you have seen one PPO, you have seen one PPO." With more and more hybrid HMOs, the same could almost be said about HMOs. Thus, the variety of HMOs and PPOs makes it difficult to make clear-cut comparisons between the two groups. There are usually some exceptions to any generalization. Nevertheless, important and significant differences exist which affect the cost-containing potential of each and the attractiveness of each to employers and employees.

### Growth Rates and Market Shares

Both HMOs and PPOs have grown at rapid rates during the 1980s. There has been over a three hundred percent increase in the growth of each since the start of the decade. Indeed, many of the same factors have contributed to the growth of each. And as noted earlier, the rapid growth of HMOs contributed to the even more rapid growth of PPOs. In recent years, the growth of each has slowed, with PPOs continuing to grow faster than HMOs. Today over 33 million Americans (employees and dependents) are enrolled in HMOs, and over 40 million citizens and their families are covered by PPOs.

During 1989, PPOs had 16 percent of employee coverage while HMOs had 17 percent. Conventional insurance covered the remaining workers. Both have highest market penetrations in the West and North Central regions. However, the Northeast is particularly unfavorable for PPOs while the South is the least supportive region for HMOs (Gabel et al. 1990).

Perhaps the chief difference between most HMOs and PPOs is that HMOs and their providers share the risk in delivering health care to an enrolled population. Most PPO providers do not engage in risk sharing. While this difference may be the primary appeal of PPOs to providers, it is also the primary reason why PPOs may not be as effective as HMOs in controlling health care costs over the long term.

Most doctors in HMOs are compensated through a capitation formula or through risk-pools (see Chapter 6). As a result, HMO providers have some financial self-interest in controlling utilization. On the other hand, PPO providers, who generally receive discounted fees for each service provided, have a financial incentive to increase utilization. Much of the inflationary effect of a fee-for-service reimbursement system remains in PPOs.

### Choice of Providers

The choice of providers is generally greater in PPOs than in HMOs. Indeed, a primary attraction of PPOs to consumers is the ability to select a provider at the point of service. In contrast, most HMO members must decide which providers they want during the period of enrollment, not at the point of service. Therefore, the HMO member is more or less committed to using the HMO providers for a designated period of time unless they wish to pay for an outside provider.

This limitation of choice in an HMO probably contributes to greater cost-containment. When an individual decides during an enrollment period whether to join an HMO, the decision is significantly affected by cost comparisons. On the other hand, when the choice of provider is made at the point-of-service, the individual is sick and cost is a lesser concern. Indeed, the more serious the case and thus the more potentially expensive, the less likely the patient's primary concern will be cost. Thus, it is not surprising that PPO enrollees are most likely

**Table 9.1**
**Monthly Cost Comparisons Among Plans in 1989 for Family Coverage**

| | Family Premium | Employer's Percent | Employer's Payment |
|---|---|---|---|
| PPOs | $271 | 71% | $192 |
| Conventional Plans with Preadmission Certification | $264 | 73% | $193 |
| HMO/IPAs | $272 | 73% | $199 |
| HMO/Staff and Group Models | $261 | 79% | $206 |

*Source*: Jon Gabel et al. ''Employer-Sponsored Health Insurance in 1989.'' *Health Affairs* 9 (Fall 1990): 161-175.

to use non-PPO providers in the more serious cases and to use the PPO for minor problems.

## Screening of Providers

HMOs, particularly staff, group, and network-model HMOs, screen providers more seriously than do most PPOs. This is something of a paradox in that a central element of the PPO concept is that more efficient providers will be selected. Yet as we have seen, PPOs do very little claims analysis of individual physicians before they contract with them. The main motivation of many PPOs is to contract with as many doctors as possible in as many locations as possible in order to enhance the PPO's marketing position. As was noted earlier, discounts do not necessarily equal efficiency. Indeed, doctors most willing to offer discounts may be those with the least business. This could indicate that their fees were too high, their quality too low, their practices were just beginning, or all of these. In any case, propensity to offer discounts does not necessarily indicate efficiency or quality.

HMOs which provide salaries to doctors must be more concerned about whom they employ. Likewise, groups of doctors who form an HMO and who share both a risk pool and a reputation will probably be more concerned about who is admitted into the group.

## Premiums

In 1989, premiums for conventional plans in both HMOs and PPOs were very similar as noted in Tables 9.1 and 9.2. The PPO family premium was the lowest for the employer although the total premium was not the lowest. Certainly the HMO costs were very competitive with the PPO charges. Moreover, between

**Table 9.2**
**Monthly Cost Comparisons Among Plans in 1989 for Individual Coverage**

| | Individual Premium | Employer's Percent | Employer's Payment |
|---|---|---|---|
| HMO/IPA | $108 | 83% | $ 90 |
| Conventional Plans with Preadmission Certification | $115 | 86% | $ 99 |
| PPO | $119 | 89% | $106 |
| HMO/Staff Group | $124 | 89% | $110 |

*Source*: Jon Gabel et al. "Employer-Sponsored Health Insurance in 1989." *Health Affairs* 9 (Fall 1990): 161-175.

1987 and 1989, the premium increases for PPOs averaged between 17 and 18 percent which were several percentage points higher than the averages for HMOs.

### Benefits

As noted in Table 9.3, benefits were similar in both HMOs and PPOs. However, HMOs tended to cover more benefits than did PPOs. Both covered more than the conventional plans.

### Utilization Review

Utilization review tends to occur more frequently in HMOs than PPOs. This is paradoxical in that utilization review is probably more critical for containing costs in a PPO than in an HMO. Since HMOs use risk-sharing, and because they take greater care in selecting providers, they have less need to rely upon utilization review to control costs. Conversely, PPOs who do not place providers at risk and who are not particularly selective in recruiting doctors, need utilization review to control costs.

While PPOs do not employ utilization review as much as HMOs, they do use some controls extensively. For example, 85 percent of PPOs have preadmission certification and 79 percent have concurrent utilization review. About half have mandatory second opinions for surgery. One potential problem with utilization review administered by PPOs is that it may not always extend to nonpreferred hospitals and physicians. Preadmission certification generally covers nonpreferred hospitals, but concurrent review may not (Gabel et al. 1987).

### Favorable Selection

Much more research has been completed on the possibility of biased selection into HMOs than has been done on PPOs. Nevertheless, the small research that

**Table 9.3**
**Comparison of Selected Benefits Among Different Plans in 1989: Percentage of Enrollees Receiving Benefits**

| Benefit | Conventional Plan | PPO | IPA HMO | Group/ Staff HMO |
|---|---|---|---|---|
| Adult Physical Exam | 34% | 42% | 95% | 99% |
| Well-Baby Care | 50% | 62% | 98% | 99% |
| Preventive Diagnostic Care | 67% | 71% | 94% | 100% |
| Home Health Care | 73% | 75% | 90% | 88% |
| Mental Health | | | | |
| Outpatient | 90% | 91% | 98% | 99% |
| Inpatient | 95% | 95% | 99% | 97% |
| Drug Treatment | 85% | 88% | 95% | 98% |
| Alcohol Treatment | 86% | 87% | 96% | 98% |
| General Dental Care | 37% | 39% | 17% | 11% |

*Source*: Jon Gabel et al. "Employer-Sponsored Health Insurance in 1989." *Health Affairs* 9 (Fall 1990): 161-175.

does exist on biased selection into PPOs indicates that the same kind of favorable selection occurs in PPOs as in HMOs. As we saw in Chapter 3, HMOs tend to attract younger, healthier employees who do not have long-standing ties with a physician. Similar employees are also the most likely to use PPO providers.

It could be that employees with established provider ties may find it more difficult to use a PPO provider than to join an HMO. Individuals join an HMO during an enrollment period that is generally open for a few weeks during only one time in the year. Thus, the choice of care occurs only one time and usually when medical care is not needed immediately. Hence, a more dispassionate, economical approach may be utilized in making the decision. The choice of plan and choice of provider are removed from each other in time.

On the other hand, PPOs present this choice of providers every time medical care is sought. Since the decision is made each time care is needed, the arrangement magnifies the emotional impact of switching providers, especially for major medical problems (Hester et al. 1987). Under such circumstances, it is very likely that the sick patient will not change providers. Therefore, it is conceivable that the choice at point of service in PPOs could produce even more favorable selection in PPOs than in HMOs.

### Employer Satisfaction

Recent surveys indicate that about 75 percent of employers are either "very" or "somewhat" satisfied with the overall performance of both their HMOs and PPOs (Gabel et al. 1990). Yet, recent double digit increases in both PPO and HMO premiums have affected employers' beliefs that the plans could control costs. This loss of confidence appears most noticeable for HMOs. Satisfaction with the cost of IPA-model HMOs fell from 86 percent to 58 percent, and for group/staff HMOs, satisfaction fell from 83 percent to 59 percent. In contrast, satisfaction with the cost of PPOs fell from 68 percent to 60 percent (Gabel et al. 1990).

Perhaps the main reason for employers' recent skepticism of HMOs is the belief that they enroll healthier employees. In a recent poll, nearly 40 percent of employee benefits managers viewed IPA enrollees as healthier than employees in conventional plans, and over 25 percent viewed their group/staff HMO enrollees as healthier (Gabel et al. 1988). In contrast, fewer than 10 percent viewed their PPO enrollees as healthier.

Most employers may not be aware of the research on biased selection by PPOs which indicates that PPOs, like HMOs, also attract healthier people. In addition, employers may be upset with the mandate requirements of HMOs. Moreover, employers generally dislike the community rating system often used by HMOs. Many may have been frustrated by HMOs' unwillingness or inability to provide experience-based ratings. For example, 30 percent of employers in a recent survey were dissatisfied with HMOs' ability to negotiate fair prices. However, only 10 percent expressed similar dissatisfaction with PPOs (Rice et al. 1989).

In any case, many employers believe that healthier employees have been attracted into HMOs, and that employers have been forced by federal equal payment provisions to make equal contributions to their HMOs and conventional plans. Some of these concerns may subside as more HMOs move to experience-based ratings.

Since employers often have had less experience with PPOs, they have had less opportunity to see that reality did not meet their expectations of PPOs. In addition, there has been no requirement for mandating equal contributions, or community ratings in PPOs.

### Employee Satisfaction

Employees are equally satisfied with access to providers in both HMOs and PPOs. Indeed, about 80 percent of employees in a recent survey were satisfied with (1) appointment wait, (2) office wait time, and (3) 24-hour access to a physician (Gabel et al. 1988). However, there were significant differences in their satisfaction with the costs and benefits of HMOs and PPOs. Approximately 75 percent of all HMO enrollees were "highly satisfied" with the cost and benefits of their HMO plan. In contrast, about 45 percent of all PPO enrollees were "highly satisfied" with the cost and benefits of their plans (Gabel et al. 1988).

As noted in Tables 9.1 and 9.2, the portion of the premiums paid by employees for family coverage were less for HMOs than for PPOs. Indeed, the employee payment for PPOs was 42 percent higher than for the staff/group-model HMOs ($79 versus $55). Yet as seen in Table 9.3, the benefits were higher in HMOs. Thus, perhaps it should not be too surprising that employees enrolled in HMOs tend to like them. The HMOs provided more benefits and charged lower premiums.

## FUTURE OF PPOs

The future of PPOs can best be predicted from their evolution and development during the last decade. At first, PPOs were primarily concerned about obtaining discounts from providers and marketing their products. With time, they have become somewhat more concerned about selecting and retaining the more efficient providers in order to control costs. In addition, they have become very involved in utilization review because it is essential if PPOs are to control costs. Likewise, PPOs in the future will develop more internal administrative controls, provider selection criteria, utilization review procedures, and management information systems to achieve cost savings (Boland 1987).

The PPO is relatively simple in its basic concept but is very difficult to implement well (Hester et al. 1987). In part, this is because PPOs do not have internal, inherent incentives to accomplish their primary goal which is to reduce health care costs. The missing incentive is risk-sharing. Without risk-sharing, PPOs are dependent on an elaborate web of thousands of contracts and discounts with individual providers, on a management information system that must trace many, many claims, and on a utilization review process which must accomplish all of the cost-containment goals of the organization. As a PPO spreads over a larger geographical area with more and more dispersed employees and providers, the more herculean the task of cost-containment becomes.

Given the above difficulties, PPOs will probably evolve toward a hybrid form that will be quite similar to the open, IPA-model HMO. More PPOs will move to adopt forms of risk-sharing arrangements with providers (capitated physician payments, gatekeeper systems, per-diem payments, and DRG-type reimbursements). PPOs may also use discounts to develop shared-risk pools for providers. Then if utilization targets are achieved, the providers can share in the risk pool. Also, PPOs will move toward greater review of provider claims and more physician profiling in order to select and keep only the efficient providers.

PPOs will probably try harder to direct employees to selected providers by increasing the coinsurance for non-preferred providers. In essence, the higher coinsurance rates may transform many PPOs into almost exclusive provider organizations. With these changes, the PPOs and HMOs will begin to appear more and more similar.

# 10

# Future HMOs and Cost Containment

## RESULTS OF COST CONTAINMENT IN THE 1980s

As noted in the introduction to this book, there are two basic approaches to controlling health care costs—regulation and competition. At the regulation end of the regulation-competition continuum, government regulates health care markets by controlling entry of providers, establishing fees, capitation, or salary, acting as sole payer, and controlling quality of care. At the opposite or competition end of the continuum, government involvement is minimal, and it is hoped that a competitive market of many independent providers seeking their own ends and establishing their own fees will control costs while also delivering quality care.

During the last decade, government has basically tried to use the competitive approach to contain health care costs, and HMOs have been part of this competition strategy. We have seen that HMOs have reduced hospital utilization. Most of this reduction is a result of reduced admissions rather than shorter lengths-of-stay. Reduced hospitalization has resulted in some hospital cost reductions, although these have not been as great as the reductions in utilization. HMOs have been less effective in controlling ambulatory utilization and costs.

We also have seen that many of the fears concerning the quality of care in HMOs are probably unfounded. Whether judged by process, structural or outcome quality measures, HMOs appear to offer care at least as good and often better than that provided by the FFS sector. Moreover, satisfaction surveys of HMO enrollees reveal that all kinds and types of enrollees have high satisfaction with their overall care in HMOs.

Thus, HMOs have considerable potential to reduce costs while maintaining quality. Has this potential been realized during the last decade? Has this competitive approach worked? While there have been some successes, the major victory of dramatic cost-containment remains elusive.

From 1976 through 1987, medical care spending increased by almost 80 percent above the general inflation rate. For Blue Cross and Blue Shield subscribers, the number of inpatient days fell 26 percent between 1981 and 1987, but the cost per day increased by 77 percent (Bodenheimer 1989). During the same time, the number of outpatient visits per subscriber increased 26 percent, while the cost per visit jumped 88 percent (Bodenheimer 1989). Likewise, physicians' fees have continued to increase faster than the general rate of inflation.

Spending on national health expenditures has more than doubled since 1980. Health care expenditures accounted for just over 9 percent of the GNP in 1980 and over 11 percent in 1990 (Levit et al. 1989). Thus, total health care costs have continued to exceed general inflation.

Why have these increases occurred during the same time that we have heard so much talk about health care cost containment? Basically, the increases have continued because the payers (employers and government) have not aggressively tackled the problem. During the 1980s, benefits continued to expand. The number of covered services offered by employers was much greater in 1985 than in 1980 (Jensen et al. 1987). For example, stop-loss coverage was more common and lifetime benefit limits rose substantially. Moreover, there has been increased coverage for chemical dependency, vision, dental, and hearing care, physical exams, home health and hospice care, and extended care services. While deductibles have increased, it is not clear that they have significantly increased more than general inflation rates. The employee's portion of coinsurance has remained basically the same.

Government has encouraged employers to be generous. Employers' payments for their employees' health care are not taxed as income for employees. Thus, as employees balance their desire for more wages versus more health care coverage, the tax benefits may tip the balance in favor of health care. Also, flexible spending accounts that allow health care costs to be paid with employees' pretax dollars also encourage greater health care expenditures.

The bottom line appears to be that workers apparently value very generous health care coverage and thus their employers provide it (Jensen et al. 1987). If employers are able to replace wage increases with higher health care premiums, and if employees accept this substitution, then health care costs will continue to advance at rates greater than general inflation. On the other hand, if employees are unwilling to give up sizable portions of their wage increases for health care coverage, and if employers are willing to be much more aggressive in their efforts to control health care costs, then cost containment may acquire real "teeth," the primary of which may be HMOs. Without these changes in the motivation and behavior of employees and employers, however, it is doubtful that HMOs will be much more than marginally useful brakes on the general inflationary trend in health care costs.

## EMPLOYERS AS SPONSORS IN AN ERA OF MANAGED COMPETITION

Alain Enthoven (1988) is the primary advocate of what he describes as "managed competition" in health care markets. If competition is to control health care costs and assure quality care, Enthoven believes that competition must be managed by sponsors who have sufficient information, clout, and self-interest to make informed and reasonable decisions when purchasing health care. Enthoven views employers, particularly large ones, as the primary sponsors for their many employees. He urges much more aggressive action by employers to control cost increases.

A more aggressive stance might encompass a number of issues including enrollment in health care plans, prices, and benefits offered by health plans, and monitoring of health care delivery by the plans.

From a cost-effective perspective, most employers are probably offering too many options and benefit packages to their employees. As a result, administrative costs and confusion are significantly increased, the employer has little focused purchasing power because employees are spread across several plans and options, and it is difficult to fix accountability for results. Most importantly, many options and vendors exacerbate the problem of favorable selection and encourage HMOs and other plans to waste resources on marketing strategies designed to attract the healthier employees. Thus, employers should dramatically reduce the number of options available to their employees.

A triple-option plan that includes a PPO, an HMO, and a regular indemnity plan might be selected which would contract to offer care to all employees for an agreed premium per employee. Employees could select which option they preferred. Such an arrangement eliminates concern about favorable selection, and it is in the plan's interest to guide employees into the most efficient option.

An even better way may be for the employer to sole source all health care with only one HMO. Of course, such a path may encounter considerable objections from employees if their favorite providers and hospitals are not in the HMO. Therefore, a point-of-service indemnity plan option might also be provided but with sufficiently high coinsurance, copayments, and deductibles to discourage its use.

The more an employer channels a large number of employees to a limited panel of providers, the greater the employer's chances of negotiating a favorable contract. Likewise, it will be easier to administer and monitor the contract. Of course, the more an employer guides employees to a select group of providers, the less freedom employees have to choose their own. This will generate considerable employee opposition. However, if employers intend to aggressively pursue cost containment, they must be prepared to meet and deflect employee resistance.

There will be much less employee opposition to an HMO if there is a good match between the HMO and the employer with respect to location, perceived image and services provided (Wrightson 1990). Primary care must be accessible with outpatient clinics in areas where employees live.

If an employer opts for sole sourcing or a total replacement approach, the employer must stress good planning for the transition period and give much thought to the type of communication and education program that will be used to explain and "sell" the new plan. Orientation sessions and "hot lines" should be used extensively to explain the benefits of the new approach.

Another step in a more aggressive stance by employers is to offer a standard benefit package and ask HMOs to submit bids only for the standard package (Enthoven 1988). Only in this way can employers make valid comparisons among bids. Moreover, a standard package is even more important if several HMOs are offered. As we have seen, HMOs can use benefit packages as a way to encourage favorable selection (e.g., wellness programs to attract younger, healthier enrollees).

If there are multiple plans or options, employers must become much more concerned about the enrollment process. Indeed, employers should present the options to the employees, enroll them, and then notify the plans as to which employees have enrolled in which plans (Enthoven 1988). When the employer provides side-by-side comparisons of different plans, the employee is in a much better position to make an informed choice. Moreover, the employer can more nearly prevent any attempt at favorable selection during the enrollment process.

Employers moving aggressively to control costs will also insist on experience-based rating from HMOs. After the 1988 Amendments to the HMO Act, all HMOs are permitted to use a form of experience-based rating. Moreover, employers must seek much more information from HMOs concerning the assumptions and calculations used by the HMOs when risk-rating of the employer's employees.

Finally, employers must become much more involved in monitoring health care delivery by HMOs. They must insist that quality assurance processes are used. In addition, they must review and analyze disenrollment. Similarly, they must review all grievances. The employer's responsibility to assure quality becomes even larger whenever a single HMO is providing health care.

## SUCCESSFUL HMOs IN AN ERA OF MANAGED COMPETITION

If employers' decide to act much more aggressively to control health care costs, some HMOs will be more successful than others in this new era of managed competition. The most successful HMOs in this environment will share several common elements including ability to offer competitive, innovative products; significant risk-sharing with providers; proficient management information systems; and success in recruiting and educating cost efficient physicians who deliver quality care.

### Competitive, Innovative Products and Successful HMOs

In the future, HMOs must be prepared to offer innovative products which employers will request. For example, employers, particularly larger companies, will demand more experience-based ratings. With the 1988 Amendments to the HMO Act, even federally-qualified HMOs may offer experience-based ratings in the form of adjusted community rating. If HMOs resist experience-based rating, they will be unable to compete for large employer groups that have predominantly younger, healthier employees (i.e., high tech firms). As a result, HMOs could lose healthy groups to experience-based indemnity insurers whose lower experience-based premiums will attract a higher proportion of the healthy groups and enrollees in a market.

If HMOs hope to resolve employers' concerns about biased selection, they must offer more experience-based ratings as well as offer products that allow one plan to offer all options to a firm's employees. Thus, the complexity, confusion, and costs associated with multiple vendors is avoided.

To accomplish this end, HMOs must be part of triple option plans or be able to offer an open-ended, point of service option that allows employees to use non-HMO providers. However, the HMO must structure the deductibles and copayments to keep use of non-HMO providers to an absolute minimum.

If HMOs wish to compete with indemnity insurers, PPOs and other providers, they must be prepared to offer more cost-sharing arrangements (higher copayments and deductibles). Such arrangements could increase direct revenues which would offset expenses and lower premiums. In addition, higher copays and deductibles tend to lower utilization. Higher cost-sharing might be particularly appropriate for inpatient services and/or outpatient mental health, emergency room visits, and other outpatient services.

With greater cost sharing, HMOs can better compete for healthier groups that do not expect to use much health care, and thus prefer the combination of lower premiums and higher cost-sharing. Similarly, greater cost sharing will allow HMOs to market less expensive plans to small companies which typically have less generous health benefits than large employers (Feldman et al. 1989).

### Risk-Sharing and Successful HMOs

The most successful HMOs in controlling costs will be those who structure real, substantive risk-sharing with their providers. It is not realistic to believe that significant efficiencies of production will be developed in medical care. It is a very labor-intensive industry similar to other high service, high labor industries, where greater productivity is often elusive. New medical discoveries and technologies often create higher costs rather than reduce total expenditures. Even if new technology did reduce unit costs of medical care, if many more units are delivered, the total cost of care will continue to escalate. The real savings in medical care costs in recent years have generally occurred, and probably will continue to occur, as a result of reduced utilization.

As we have seen, HMOs use several strategies such as risk-sharing and utilization review to control utilization of health care. However, utilization review has only limited effectiveness. Moreover, it is expensive and does not have a linear relationship to savings (e.g., every extra dollar spent on utilization review will not necessarily save a dollar).

Utilization review has been most successful in reducing hospitalization. While HMOs and employers may be able to obtain better rates from hospitals, it is doubtful that they can accomplish dramatic, additional reduced utilization in hospitals from utilization review. The area of greatest growth in utilization and cost increases in recent years has been in outpatient services and in physician services and fees. Yet, these activities, because of their decentralized and numerous nature, are much less susceptible to the constraining influence of utilization review. Moreover, utilization review of these activities demands more resources and is more expensive. Thus, if real savings are to occur in the outpatient/physician services areas, the pernicious effects of fee-for-service must be reduced, and provider risk-sharing is the most potent remedy.

Capitation is already a widely accepted method of payment in HMOs and the more successful HMOs will expand its use. Clearly, capitation (as compared to FFS) encourages a more conservative (some say too conservative) approach to medical practice.

The size of risk pools and the amount of "withholds" are very important variables in HMOs' risk-sharing strategies (Welch et al. 1990). If the risk pools are too large, no single physician will feel as though his or her actions have much impact on the pool. However, if only one physician's patients form a risk pool, the incentive to underutilize may be too strong.

Risk pools involving subgroups of physicians in an HMO average 34 primary-care physicians' while pools covering an entire HMO may include hundreds of physicians (Welch et al. 1990). There is obviously very little risk involved in pools of several hundred physicians. Even in an average subgroup pool of 34 physicians, any single physician is responsible for only 3 percent (one thirty-fourth) of any additional costs he or she generates. This is not much of an incentive or disincentive. More successful HMOs will, after trial and error, find a pool size that will be small enough to encourage each individual physician to recognize that his or her behavior will directly and significantly affect the pool, yet not be so small as to encourage harmful underutilization.

From a cost containment perspective, a pool covering a single physician's patients generates the greatest incentive to conserve medical care. However, relatively few (less than 20 percent) HMOs place individual physicians at risk today (Welch et al. 1990). Such pools pose real threats to quality as noted in Chapter 6. HMOs can move to much smaller risk pools than we see today without adopting the single physician pools.

In a pool of five to ten physicians, each would recognize their individual impact on the group pool. Just as importantly, each would see and feel directly the impact of colleagues actions' on the pool's funds. Such pools would be most effective in a medical group structure with established group practice norms and informal and formal mechanisms to control both utilization and quality. In such an environment, each physician is reviewing the quality and efficiency of his colleague's practice.

The size of the withhold is another factor determining the level of risk felt by providers. Since most withholds are less than 20 percent today, it is doubtful that they have a very significant impact on physician behavior. In the future, HMOs that wish to have a greater impact on their physicians' practice patterns may need to consider larger withholds (at least 20 percent or larger). As the size of the withholds increase, and as the number in the risk pools decrease, HMOs will have a more profound effect on providers' behavior.

The method of payment (capitation versus FFS), the size of risk pools, and the amount of the withholds will matter little if few HMO patients are in a physician's practice. Physicians participating in HMOs today receive an average of only 30 percent of their income from HMOs (Rosenbach et al. 1988). This average is often too low for HMOs to have a significant influence over their physicians' practice patterns. Successful HMOs in the future will increase this average by attracting more enrollees and/or by carefully winnowing its providers to maintain those who most value cost-effective, quality care.

### Management Information Systems and Successful HMOs

There are several reasons why successful HMOs must have better management information systems (MIS) in the future. First, employers will seek more experience-based ratings from HMOs. In the past, most HMOs developed a community rating that applied to all enrollees in the plan. Moreover, since HMOs received payment according to a per capita formula and often paid providers by salary or capitation, there was less need to keep utilization or claims data for each individual enrollee. However, the push from employers for experience-based ratings will require that successful HMOs be able to document actual use by a firm's employees. This will place much greater pressure on HMOs' data processing and analytical systems, and its underwriting and actuarial personnel and units.

HMOs that develop their management information systems and move to experience-based ratings, will be better able to predict how the loss of a particular group of enrollees, or the addition of another group will affect the HMO's need to provide services. Thus, the HMO with experience-based data is better able to quickly respond to changes in enrollment. In contrast, the HMO using community rating and without a good MIS may not know how the withdrawal or addition of a particular group may affect its operations and its premiums until long after the change has occurred. Of course, by then it may already be too late (Wrightson 1990).

Likewise, HMOs' increasing use of capitation to reimburse providers places greater pressure on the same MIS and underwriting units. The capitation fee is based on projections of use for different subgroups of enrollees. Thus, HMOs must develop capitation formula that accurately predict the utilization of these various groups and that compensate for adverse or favorable selection. Indeed, smaller risk-pools (which may be used to increase risk-sharing by providers) will demand even more sensitive and accurate capitation formula.

Successful HMOs' cost containment and quality assurance processes will also require better management information systems. As HMOs' cost containment efforts expand from hospitals to outpatient and physicians' services, successful HMOs must be better able to monitor services provided by individual doctors. Outliers must be identified and their behavior changed. The MIS will become an integral part of the educational efforts and physician profiling provided by the HMO to its providers. Those providers who resist change and who remain persistent outliers will be removed from the plan. The MIS will provide the documentation to support such action.

As HMOs encourage their providers to engage in increased risk-sharing, the danger of underutilization or loss of quality will increase. Thus, HMOs will also need good management information systems to monitor quality criteria among providers and to identify outliers.

## Recruitment and Orientation of Physicians in Successful HMOs

A critical factor in any successful HMO will be its ability to recruit and retain quality, cost conscious physicians. Successful HMOs in the future will use greater care in recruiting and selecting physicians who are comfortable with the HMO concept and who believe that quality care can be offered through HMOs.

HMOs will seek good relations with providers by involving physicians as key members of the management team and by assuring that physicians are involved in peer utilization and quality review processes. Successful HMOs will provide doctors timely feedback of practice and utilization data.

Successful HMOs will develop small provider risk-sharing pools into informal peer review groups which can oversee their own members in terms of utilization and quality assurance. This can happen if the groups are more than just isolated members of a common risk-pool who otherwise have little communication with one another.

If HMOs bring the members of small risk pools together frequently, and provide them with utilization and quality assurance data, then they can develop informal norms that will well serve the interests of the group and the HMO. In addition, successful HMOs will assure physician support by eliminating as many bureaucratic hassles and as much paperwork as possible, and by assuring adequate support staff in order that physicians can practice medicine as opposed to completing other tasks (Topping and Fottler 1990).

## THREATS TO QUALITY IN AN ERA OF MANAGED HEALTH CARE COMPETITION

The chief threats to quality under managed health care competition is that citizens will lose some of their freedom to select providers and some of their access to care. Undoubtedly, there is some trade-off between containing cost increases and unlimited choice of providers. It is difficult to have completely wide open and equal access to all possible providers while also containing costs.

We should also remember that some limits on choice of provider do not equal complete loss-of-freedom to select a doctor. Enrollees in HMOs would continue to have a wide selection of HMO providers. In addition, if enrollees wished to pay much larger copayments and deductibles, they could still use non-HMO providers.

Concerns about access to care should be softened by the considerable body of research, as noted in prior chapters of this book, which indicates that most enrollees are very satisfied with access to care in HMOs. It is also well to remember that as long as everyone receives as much medical care as they desire, rather than what they need, cost containment will remain an elusive goal.

As we saw in Chapter 6, there is wide variation in medical practice patterns among doctors. Some practice aggressive medicine while others are more conservative. Yet, evidence does not indicate that the health outcomes or health status of a population varies with its doctors' practice patterns. In fact, too many services may increase not only cost but risk (Luft 1982).

Most research on structural, process, and outcome measures of quality indicate that HMOs provide quality care that equals if not exceeds that provided by the FFS sector. Moreover, HMO enrollees appear to be very satisfied with the quality of their care. Of course, as competition increases in a managed care environment, and as physicians experience more intense risk-sharing, they may be more predisposed to guard the economic bottom line. These possible tendencies point to the great need for successful HMOs to have effective and comprehensive quality assurance processes. These procedures can help assure adequate health care while also guarding the HMO against possible malpractice lawsuits. Moreover, such procedures enhance an HMO's marketing efforts. Thus, assuring quality will be economically as well as ethically attractive.

## WILL MANAGED COMPETITION CONTROL HEALTH CARE COST INCREASES?

After looking at the increases of health care costs over the last thirty years, one should not be particularly optimistic that "managed competition" will hold health care cost increases below the general rate of inflation. The chances of "managed competition" and HMOs successfully containing health care costs are probably less than 50/50. Indeed, it is possible that most Americans are not too concerned about the cost of health care. A recent Gallup survey reveals that three out of four Americans believe that the United States should spend *more*, not less of the total national budget on health care (''Poll Shows Mood to Spend on Health'' 1990).

Of course, if government spends more on health care without raising taxes, it must spend less on education, transportation, housing, environment, and other values that contribute to our quality of life. Moreover, our major competitors in Japan and Germany spend considerably less of their GNP on health care, yet they are as healthy as we. If American employers must spend more on health care without raising the prices of their products, they must either reduce their employees' wages or become less competitive.

Thus, if we follow our thirty year path of spending an ever-increasing share of our GNP on health services, then we risk becoming a less competitive nation even as we fail to significantly improve our health. Surely such a possibility should increase our hopes that HMOs have the potential, within an environment of managed competition, to control health care cost increases. For if they fail to do so, a much more centralized, regulated, and government-dominated approach to health care cost containment lies ahead. As Pogo said, ''Man never reads the writing on the wall until his back is against it.'' As regards health care costs, our backs may be getting close to the wall.

# Bibliography


Aaron, H., and W. B. Schwartz. "Rationing Health Care: The Choice Before Us." *Science* 247 (1990): 418–422.

Abel-Smith, B. *Cost Containment in Health Care: A Study of 12 European Countries, 1977–1983*. London: Bedford Square Press of the National Council for Voluntary Organizations, 1984.

Accreditation Association for Ambulatory Care. *Accreditation Handbook for Ambulatory Health Care: 1989–90*. Skokie, IL: Accreditation Association for Ambulatory Health Care, Inc., 1989.

Altman, S. H., and M. A. Rodwin. "Halfway Competitive Markets and Ineffective Regulation: The American Health Care System." *Journal of Health Politics, Policy and Law* 13 (1988): 323–339.

Anderson, G., and J. Knickman. "Adverse Selection Under a Voucher System: Grouping Medicare Recipients by Level of Expenditure." *Inquiry* 21 (1984): 135–143.

Anderson, G., and E. Steinberg. "Predicting Hospital Readmissions in the Medicare Population." *Inquiry* 22 (1985): 251–258.

Anderson, G. F., E. P. Steinberg, J. Holloway, and J. C. Cantor. "Paying for HMO Care: Issues and Options In Setting Capitation Rates." *Milbank Quarterly* 64 (1986): 548–565.

Anderson, J., A. L. Resnick, and P. M. Gertman. *Prediction of Subsequent Year Reimbursement Using the Medicare History Files: II. A Comparison of Several Models*. Boston: Boston University Medical Center, University Health Policy Consortium, 1983.

Anderson, M. D., and P. D. Fox. "Lessons From Medicaid Managed Care." *Health Affairs* 6 (1987): 71–86.

Anderson, O. W., T. E. Herold, B. W. Butler, C. H. Kohrman, and E. M. Morrison. *HMO Development: Patterns and Prospects*. Chicago: Pluribus Press, 1985.

Andrews, R. M., B. A. Curbow, E. Owen, and A. Burke. "The Effects of Method of Presenting Health Plan Information on HMO Enrollment by Medicaid Beneficiaries." *Health Services Research* 24 (1989): 311–327.

Barger, S. B., D. G. Hillman, and H. R. Garland. *The PPO Handbook*. Rockville, MD: Aspen Publications, 1985.

Bates, E. and B. Brown. "Geriatric Care Needs and HMO Technology: A Theoretical Analysis and Initial Findings From the National Medicare Competition Evaluations." *Medical Care* 26 (1988): 488–498.

Beebe, J., J. Lubitz, and P. Eggers. "Using Prior Utilization to Determine Payments for Medicare Enrollees in Health Maintenance Organizations." *Health Care Financing Review* 6 (1985): 27–38.

Berki, S. E., and M.L.F. Ashcraft. "HMO Enrollment: Who Joins What and Why: A Review of the Literature." *Milbank Memorial Fund Quarterly* 58 (1980): 588–632.

Berki, S. E., M.L.F. Ashcraft, R. Penchansky, and R. S. Fortus. "Enrollment Choice in a Multi-HMO Setting: The Roles of Health Risk, Financial Vulnerability and Access to Care." *Medical Care* 15 (1977): 95–114.

Bernton, C. T. "What is the Future for Health Promotion in HMOs?" *American Journal of Health Promotion* (Spring 1987).

Berwick, D. W. "Monitoring Quality in HMOs." *Business and Health* 5 (November 1987): 9–12.

Bice, T. W. "Risk Vulnerability and Enrollment in a Prepaid Group Practice." *Medical Care* 13 (1975): 698–703.

Billett, T. C., and J. A. Cantor. "Employer's Experience with Preferred Provider Organizations." *Compensation and Benefits Management* (Autumn 1985): 21–26.

Blendon, R. J., R. Leitman, I. Morrison, and K. Donelson. "Satisfaction with Health Systems in Ten Nations." *Health Affairs* 9 (1990): 185–192.

Blue Cross and Blue Shield Association. "Survey Shows HMO Members Happy With Quality of Care." *Medical Benefits* 6 (April 1989): 3.

Bodenheimer, T. S. "Payment Mechanisms Under a National Health Program." *Medical Care Review* 46 (1989): 3–43.

Boland, P. "Trends in Second-Generation PPOs." *Health Affairs* 4 (1987): 75–81.

Bonanno, J. B., and T. Wetle. "HMO Enrollment of Medicare Recipients: An Analysis of Incentives and Barriers." *Journal of Health Politics, Policy and Law* 9 (1984): 41–62.

Brook, R. H., and K. N. Lohr. "Efficacy, Effectiveness, Variations, and Quality." *Medical Care* 23 (1985): 710–722.

Brown, R. S., and K. Langwell. "Enrollment Patterns in Medicare HMOs: Implications for Access to Care." In *Advances in Health Economics and Health Services Research*, 9, eds. R. M. Scheffler and L. F. Rossiter, 69–96. Greenwich, CT: JAI Press, 1988.

Buchanan, J. L., and S. Cretin. "Risk Selection of Families Electing HMO Membership." *Medical Care* 24 (1986): 39–51.

Christianson, J. B. "Alternative Delivery Systems in Rural Areas." *Health Services Research* 23 (1989): 849–889.

Christianson, J. B. "The Impact of HMOs: Evidence and Research Issues." *Journal of Health Politics, Policy and Law* 5 (1980): 354–367.

Christianson, J. B., and M. Shadle. "HMOs in Rural Areas: Pros, Cons, and Financial

Realities.'' In *Financing Rural Health Care*, eds. L. Straub and N. Walzer, 149–173. New York: Praeger Publishers, 1988.

Christianson, J. B., M. Shadle, M. M. Hunter, S. Hartwell, and J. McGee. ''The New Environment for Rural HMOs.'' *Health Affairs* 5 (1986): 105–121.

Chiswick, B. R. ''Hospital Utilization: An Analysis of SMSA Differences in Occupancy Rates, Admission Rates and Bed Rates.'' *Explorations in Economic Research* 3 (1976): 326–378.

Citizens Fund. *Spending More and Getting Less: A Comparison of the Cost and Quality of Health Care in the United States and the World.* Washington, DC: Citizens Fund, 1990.

Columbia University School of Public Health and Administrative Medicine. *Family Medical Care Under Three Types of Health Insurance*. New York: Foundation of Employee Health, Medical Care and Welfare, Inc., 1962.

Connell, F. A., R. W. Day, and J. P. LoGerfo. ''Hospitalization of Medicaid Children: Analysis of Small Area Variations in Admission Rates.'' *American Journal of Public Health* 71 (1981): 606–613.

Danzon, P. M, W. G. Manning, and M. S. Marquis. ''Factors Influencing Laboratory Test Use and Prices.'' *Health Care Financing Review* 5 (1984) 23–32.

Davies, A. R., and J. E. Ware. ''Involving Consumers in Quality Assessment.'' *Health Affairs* 7 (1988): 33–48.

Davies, A. R., J. E. Ware, R. H. Brook, J. R. Peterson, and J. P. Newhouse. ''Consumer Acceptance of Prepaid and Fee-For-Service Medical Care: Results From a Randomized Controlled Trial.'' *Health Service Research* 3 (1986): 429.

de Lissovoy, G., T. Rice, J. Gabel, and H. Gelzer. ''Preferred Provider Organizations: One Year Later.'' *Inquiry* 24 (1987): 124–36.

DesHarnais, S. I. ''Enrollment in and Disenrollment from Health Maintenance Organizations by Medicaid Recipients.'' *Health Care Financing Review* 6 (1985): 39–50.

Diehr, P., D. Martin, R. Leickly, L. Krueger, N. Silberg, and S. Barchet. ''Use of Ambulatory Health Care Services in a Preferred Provider Organization.'' *Medical Care* 25 (1987): 1033–1043.

Diehr, P., R. Leickly, M. Tatarsky, B. Hermanson, L. Krueger, and N. Silberg. ''Use of a Preferred Provider by Employees of the Preferred Provider.'' *Health Services Research* 23 (1988): 537–554.

Donabedian, A. ''The Quality of Care in a Health Maintenance Organization.'' *Inquiry* 20 (1983): 218.

Dowd, B. and R. Feldman. ''Biased Selection in Twin Cities Health Plans.'' In *Advances in Health Economics and Health Services Research* 6, eds. R. M. Scheffler and L. F. Rossiter, 253–274. Greenwich, CT: JAI Press, 1985.

Dowd, B. E. ''HMOs and Twin Cities Admission Rates.'' *Health Services Research* 21 (1986): 177–188.

Eddy, D. M. ''Variations in Physician Practice: The Role of Uncertainty.'' *Health Affairs* 2 (1984): 74–89.

Ellis, R. P. ''The Effect of Prior-Year Health Expenditures on Health Coverage Plan Choice.'' In *Advances in Health Economics and Health Services Research* 6, eds. R. M. Scheffler and L. F. Rossiter, 149–170. Greenwich, CT: JAI Press, 1985.

Eggers, P., and R. Prihoda. ''Pre-Enrollment Reimbursement Patterns of Medicare Beneficiaries Enrolled in 'At Risk' HMOs.'' *Health Care Financing Review* 2 (1982): 55–73.

Eggers, P. ''Risk Differential Between Medicare Beneficiaries Enrolled and Not Enrolled in an HMO.'' *Health Care Financing Review* 1 (1980): 91–99.

Eisenberg, J. M. *Doctors' Decisions and the Cost of Medical Care*. Ann Arbor, MI: Health Administration Press, 1986.

Eisenberg, J. M. ''Physician Utilization: The State of Research About Physicians' Practice Patterns.'' *Medical Care* 23 (1985): 461–483.

Enthoven, A. ''Managed Competition of Alternative Delivery Systems.'' *Journal of Health Politics, Policy and Law* 13 (1988): 305–321.

Enthoven, A. C. ''Competition of Alternative Delivery Systems.'' In *Competition in the Health Care Sector: Past, Present, and Future*, proceedings of a conference sponsored by the Bureau of Economics, Federal Trade Commission (March 1978): 322–51.

Enthoven, A. C. *Health Plan: The Only Practical Solution to the Soaring Cost of Medical Care*. Reading, MA: Addison-Wesley Publishing Co., 1980.

Enthoven, A. C. ''Managed Competition in Health Care and the Unfinished Agenda.'' *Health Care Financing Review* (1986 Supplement): 105–119.

Enthoven, A., and R. Kronick. ''A Consumer-Choice Health Plan for the 1990s: Part I.'' *The New England Journal of Medicine* 320 (1989): 29–37.

Enthoven, A. and R. Kronick. ''A Consumer-Choice Health Plan for the 1990s: Part II.'' *The New England Journal of Medicine* 320 (1989): 94–101.

Epstein, A., B. Colin, and B. McNeil. ''The Use of Ambulatory Testing in Prepaid and Fee-for-Service Group Practices.'' *New England Journal of Medicine* 314 (1986): 1089–2094.

Epstein, A. M., R. M. Hortley, and J. R. Charlton. ''A Comparison of Ambulatory Test Ordering for Hypertensive Patients in the United States and England.'' *Journal of the American Medical Association* 252 (1984): 1723–26.

Evans, R. G. ''Finding the Levers, Finding the Courage: Lessons from Cost Containment in North America.'' *Journal of Health Politics, Policy and Law* 11 (1986): 585–615.

Falkson, J. L. *HMOs and the Politics of Health System Reform*. Bowie, MD: Robert J. Brady Co., 1979.

Farley, P. J., and A. C. Monheit. ''Selectivity in the Demand for Health Insurance and Health Care.'' In *Advances in Health Economics and Health Services Research* 6, eds. R. M. Scheffler and L. R. Rossiter, 231–248. Greenwich, CT: JAI Press, 1985.

Feldman, R., B. Dowd, D. McCann, and A. Johnson. ''The Competitive Impact of Health Maintenance Organizations on Hospital Finances: An Exploratory Study.'' *Journal of Health Politics, Policy and Law* 10 (1986): 675–697.

Feldman, R., J. Kralewski, and B. Dowd. ''Health Maintenance Organizations: The Beginning or the End.'' *Health Services Research* 24 (1989): 191–211.

Feldstein, P. J. ''The Effects of Utilization Review Programs on Health Care Use and Expenditures.'' *The New England Journal of Medicine* 318 (May 19, 1988): 1310–1314.

Foster Higgins. *Health Care Benefits Survey 1988*. Princeton, NJ: Foster Higgins, 1988.

Foster Higgins. *Health Care Benefits Survey 1987*. Princeton, NJ: Foster Higgins, 1987.

Fox, P. D., and L. Heinen. *Determinants of HMO Success*. Ann Arbor, MI: Health Administration Press, 1987.

Francis, A. M., L. Polissar, and A. B. Lorenz. ''Care of Patients With Colorectal Cancer: A Comparison of Health Maintenance Organization and Fee-for-Service Practices.'' *Medical Care* 22 (1984): 418–426.

Freund, D. A., and E. Neuschler. ''Overview of Medicaid Capitation and Case-Management Initiatives.'' *Health Care Financing Review* (Supplement 1986): 21–30.

Freund, D. A., L. F. Rossiter, P. D. Fox, J. A. Meyer, R. E. Hurley, T. S. Carey, and J. E. Paul. ''Evaluation of the Medicaid Competition Demonstrations.'' *Health Care Financing Review* 11 (1989): 81–97.

Fritz, D., and D. Repko. ''A Blueprint for Forging New HMO Relationships.'' *Business and Health* 3 (July/August 1986): 38–40.

Fuchs, V. R., and J. S. Hahn. ''How Does Canada Do It?'' A Comparison of Expenditures for Physicians' Services in the United States and Canada,'' *The New England Journal of Medicine* 323 (1990): 884–890.

Gabel, J., C. Jajich-Toth, G. de Lissovoy, T. Rice and H. Cohen. ''The Changing World of Group Health Insurance.'' *Health Affairs* 7 (1988): 48–65.

Gabel, J., C. Jajich-Toth, K. Williams, S. Loughran, and K. Hough. ''The Health Insurance Industry in Transition.'' *Health Affairs* 6 (1987): 46–60.

Gabel, J., D. Ermann, T. Rice, and G. de Lissovoy. ''The Emergence and Future of PPOs.'' *Journal of Health Politics, Policy and Law* 11 (1986): 305–313.

Gabel, J., S. DiCarlo, C. Sullivan and T. Rice. ''Employer-Sponsored Health Insurance 1989.'' *Health Affairs* 9 (1990): 161–175.

Garfinkel, S. A., W. E. Schlenger, K. R. McLeroy, F. A. Bryan, J. G. York, G. H. Dunteman, and A. S. Friedlob. ''Choice of Payment Plan in the Medicare Capitation Demonstration.'' *Medical Care* 24 (1986): 628–640.

Garnick, D. W., H. S. Luft, L. B. Gardner, E. M. Morrison, M. Barrett, A. O'Neil, and B. Harvey. ''Services and Charges by PPO Physicians for PPO and Indemnity Patients: An Episode of Care Comparison.'' *Medical Care* 18 (1990): 894–906.

Gaus, C., B. S. Cooper, and C. G. Hirschman. ''Contrasts in HMO and Fee-For-Service Performance.'' *Social Security Bulletin* 39 (1976): 3–14.

Gerbert, A., and W. A. Hargreaves. ''Measuring Physician Behavior.'' *Medical Care* 24 (1987): 838–847.

Ginsburg, P., S. Hosek, and M. Marquis. ''Who Joins A PPO?'' *Business and Health* 4 (February 1987): 36–38.

Gold, M. ''Physician Incentive Arrangements in Prepaid Managed Groups.'' Association of America, Conference Presentation, Washington, DC, 1988.

Gold, M., and D. Hodges. ''Health Maintenance Organizations in 1988.'' *Health Affairs* 8 (1989): 125–138.

Gold, M., M. Joffe, T. L. Kennedy, and A. M. Tucker. ''Pharmacy Benefits in Health Maintenance Organizations.'' *Health Affairs* 8 (1989): 182–190.

Goldberg, L. G., and W. Greenberg. ''The Competitive Response of Blue Cross to the Health Maintenance Organization.'' *Economic Inquiry* 18 (1980): 55–68.

Goldsmith, J. *Can Hospitals Survive*? Homewood, IL: Dow Jones-Irwin, 1981.

Goodman, L. J., and J. E. Swartwout. ''Comparative Aspects of Medical Practice.'' *Medical Care* 22 (1984): 255–267.

Greenberg, J., W. Lentz, M. Greenlick, J. Malone, S. Ervin, and D. Kodner. ''The Social HMO Demonstration: Early Experience.'' *Health Affairs* 7 (1988): 66–79.

Greenwald, H. P., M. L. Peterson, and L. P. Garrison. ''Interspecialty Variation in Office-Based Care.'' *Medical Care* 22 (1984): 14–29.

Group Health Association of America. *Annual HMO Industry Survey 1988*. Washington, DC: GHAA, 1988.

Group Health Association of America. *Financial Performance of Health Maintenance Organizations*. Washington, DC: GHAA, 1988.

Group Health Association of America. *National HMO Census Survey, 1976–1977 Summary*. Washington, DC: GHAA, 1977.

Gruber, L. R., M. Shadle, and C. L. Plich. ''From Movement to Industry: The Growth of HMOs.'' *Health Affairs* 7 (1988): 197–208.

Guterman, S., P. W. Eggers, G. Riley, T. F. Greene, and S. A. Terrell. ''The First Three Years of Medicare Prospective Payment: An Overview.'' *Health Care Financing Review* 9 (1988): 67–77.

Halvorson, G. C. *How to Cut Your Company's Health Care Costs*. Paramus, NJ: Prentice-Hall Information Services, 1988.

Ham, F. L. ''How to Check Out an HMO.'' *Business and Health* 7 (June 1989): 38–42.

Hartwell, S. *Key Issues in Rural Health Care*. Excelsior, MN: InterStudy, 1988.

Hartzema, A. G., and D. B. Christenson. ''Nonmedical Factors Associated with the Prescribing Volume Among Family Practitioners in an HMO.'' *Medical Care* 21 (1983): 990–1000.

Hays, R. D., and J. E. Ware. ''My Medical Coverage is Better Than Yours: Social Desirability and Patient Satisfaction Ratings.'' *Medical Care* 24 (1986): 519–524.

Hellinger, F. J. ''Selection Bias in Health Maintenance Organizations: Analysis of Recent Evidence.'' *Health Care Financing Review* 9 (1987): 55–63.

Hester, J., A. Wouters, and N. Wright. ''Evaluation of a Preferred Provider Organization.'' *The Milbank Quarterly* 65 (1987): 575–613.

Hetherington, R., C. E. Hopkins, and M. I. Roemer. *Health Insurance Plans: Promise and Performance*. New York: Wiley Interscience, 1975.

Hillman, A. L., M. V. Pauly, and J. J. Kerstein. ''How Do Financial Incentives Affect Physicians' Clinical Decisions and the Financial Performance of Health Maintenance Organizations?'' *New England Journal of Medicine* 321 (1989): 86–92.

''HMO/Medicare Demonstration Projects Serve Elderly Well.'' *Group Health News* 26 (1985): 1–3.

Hohlen, M. M., L. M. Manheim, G. V. Fleming, S. M. Davidson, B. K. Yudkowsky, S. M. Werner, and G. M. Wheatley. ''Access to Office-Based Physicians Under Capitation Reimbursement and Medicaid Case Management.'' *Medical Care* 28 (1990): 59–68.

Holahan, J., J. Hadley, W. Scanlon, R. Lee, and J. Bluck. ''Paying for Physician Services Under Medicare and Medicaid.'' *Milbank Memorial Fund Quarterly* 57 (1979): 183–211.

Hornbrook, M. C., and Berki, S. E. ''Practice Mode and Payment Methods: Effects on Use, Cost, Quality and Access. *Medical Care* 23 (1985): 484–508.

Hornbrook, M. C. ''Examination of the AAPCC Methodology in an HMO Prospective Payment Demographic Project.'' *Group Health Journal* 5 (1984): 13–21.

Hulka, B. S., and J. R. Wheat. ''Patterns of Utilization.'' *Medical Care* 23 (1985): 438–460.

Hurley, R. E., and D. A. Freund. "A Typology of Medicaid Managed Care." *Medical Care* 26 (1988): 764–773.

InterStudy. *The Bottom Line: HMO Premiums and Profitability: 1988–1989*. Excelsior, MN.: InterStudy, 1989.

InterStudy. *Considerations in Developing a Rural HMO*. Excelsior, MN.: InterStudy, 1988.

InterStudy. *From HMO Movement to Managed Care Industry*. Excelsior, MN.: InterStudy, 1988.

InterStudy. *The InterStudy Edge*. Excelsior, MN.: InterStudy, Spring, 1990.

InterStudy. *The InterStudy Edge*. Excelsior, MN.: InterStudy, Spring, 1989.

InterStudy. *The InterStudy Edge*. Excelsior, MN.: InterStudy, Spring, 1988.

InterStudy. *The June 1985 HMO Summary*. Excelsior, MN.: InterStudy, 1985.

InterStudy. *National HMO Census*. Excelsior, MN.: InterStudy, 1984.

InterStudy. *National HMO Census*. Excelsior, MN.: InterStudy, 1983.

InterStudy. *National HMO Census*. Excelsior, MN.: InterStudy, 1982.

InterStudy. *National HMO Census*. Excelsior, MN.: InterStudy, 1981.

InterStudy. *The 1988 January Update of Medicare Enrollment in HMOs*. Excelsior, MN.: InterStudy, 1988.

InterStudy. *The 1986 June Update*. Excelsior, MN.: InterStudy, 1986.

InterStudy. *1988 National HMO Firms*. Excelsior, MN.: InterStudy, 1988.

InterStudy. *1989 National Managed Care Firms*. Excelsior, MN.: InterStudy, 1989.

Iversen, L. H., C. L. Polich, and C. N. Oberg. "Factors Leading to Medicare Risk Contracting Success or Failure: The HMO Perspective." *GHAA Journal* (Winter 1987/1988): 30–42.

Iversen, L. H., and C. L. Polich. *1986 December Update of Medicare Enrollment in HMOs*. Excelsior, MN.: InterStudy, 1987.

Iversen, L. H., and C. L. Polich. *The Future of Medicare and HMOs*. Excelsior, MN.: InterStudy, 1985.

Iversen, L. H., C. L. Polich, J. R. Dahl, and L. J. Secord. *Improving Health and Long-Term Care for the Elderly*. Excelsior, MN.: InterStudy, 1986.

Iversen, L. H., C. N. Oberg, and C. L. Polich. "The Availability of Long-Term Care Services for Medicare Beneficiaries in Health Maintenance Organizations." *Medical Care* 26 (1988): 918–925.

Jackson-Beeck, M., and J. H. Kleinman. "Evidence for Self-Selection Among Health Maintenance Enrollees." *Journal of American Medical Association* 250 (1983): 2826–2829.

Jensen, G. A., M. A. Morrisey, and J. W. Marcus. "Cost Sharing and the Changing Pattern of Employer-Sponsored Health Benefits." *The Milbank Quarterly* 65 (1987): 521–550.

Johns, L., R. Derzon, and M. Anderson. *Selective Contracting in California*. Final Report. Washington, DC: Lewin and Associates, 1985.

Johnson, A. N., and D. Aquilina. "The Impacts of Health Maintenance Organizations and Competition on Hospitals in Minneapolis/St. Paul." *Journal of Health Politics, Policy and Law* 10 (1986): 659–674.

Johnson, R. L. "Alternative Delivery Systems to Diversify Hospital Revenues." *Topics in Health Care Financing* (Fall 1981).

Johnson and Higgins. *Corporate Health Care Benefits Survey 1986*. Princeton, NJ: Johnson and Higgins, 1986.

Joint Commission on Accreditation of Healthcare Organizations. *Quality Assurance in Managed Care Organizations*. Chicago: Joint Commission, 1989.

Juba, D., J. R. Lave, and J. Shaddy. "An Analysis of the Choice of Health Benefits Plans." *Inquiry* 17 (1980): 62–71.

Kechley Report on Health Care. "What Does Quality of Care Mean?" *Medical Benefits* (February 29, 1988): 9.

Kimmey, J. R. *A Review of Selected Provider Arrangements*. Madison, WI: Institute for Health Planning, 1983.

Kindig, D. A., H. Movassaghi, N. C. Dunham, D. I. Zwick, and C. Taylor. "Trends in Physician Availability in 10 Urban Areas from 1963 to 1980." *Inquiry* 24 (1987): 136–146.

Kirkman-Liff, B. L. "Refusal of Care: Evidence From Arizona." *Health Affairs* 4 (1985): 15–24.

Kirkman-Liff, B. L., J. B. Christianson, and T. Kirkman-Liff. "Evaluation of Arizona's Indigent Care System." *Medical Care* 6 (1987): 46–58.

Kralewski, J. E., D. D. Countryman, and L. Pitt. "Hospital and Health Maintenance Organization Financial Agreements for Inpatient Services: A Case Study of the Minneapolis/St. Paul Area." *Health Care Financing Review* 4 (1983): 79–84.

Langwell, K. M., and J. P. Hadley. "Capitation and the Medicare Program: History, Issues and Evidence." *Health Care Financing Review* (Supplement 1986): 9–20.

Langwell, K. M., and J. P. Hadley. "Evaluation of Medicare Competition Demonstrations." *Health Care Financing Review* 11 (1989): 65–80.

Langwell, K. M., and J. P. Hadley. "Insights From the Medicare HMO Demonstrations." *Medical Care* 9 (1990): 74–84.

Langwell, K., L. Rossiter, R. Brown, L. Nelson, S. Nelson, and K. Berman. "Early Experience of Health Maintenance Organizations Under Medicare Competition Demonstrations." *Health Care Financing Review* 8 (1987): 37–55.

Leal, S. "Trust Funds Determine How to Run Their Own PPO." *Business and Health* 4 (February 1987): 40–41.

Leibowitz, A., and J. L. Buchanan. "Setting Capitations for Medicaid: A Case Study." *Health Care Financing Review* 11 (1990): 79–85.

Levit, K. R., M. S. Freeland, and D. R. Waldo. "Health Spending and Ability to Pay: Business, Individuals, and Government." *Health Care Financing Review* 10 (1989): 1–11.

Lewis, K. "Comparison of Use by Enrolled and Recently Disenrolled Populations in a Health Maintenance Organization." *Health Services Research* 19 (1984): 1–22.

Lichtenstein, R., and J. W. Thomas. "Including a Measure of Health Status in Medicare's Health Maintenance Organization Capitation Formula: Reliability Issues." *Medical Care* 25 (1987): 101–110.

Linn, L. S., and M. R. DiMattro, B. L. Chang, and D. W. Cope. "Consumer Values and Subsequent Satisfaction Ratings of Physician Behavior." *Medical Care* 22 (1984): 804–812.

Linn, L. S., and S. Greenfield. "Patient Suffering and Patient Satisfaction Among the Chronically Ill." *Medical Care* 20 (1982): 425–431.

Lohr, K. N., K. D. Yordy, and S. O. Thier. "Current Issues in Quality of Care." *Health Affairs* 7 (1988): 5–18.

Louis Harris and Associates. *A Report Card on HMOs: Summary Report*. Prepared for the Henry J. Kaiser Family Foundation, 1984.

Lubitz, J., J. Beebe, and G. Riley. ''Improving the Medicare HMO Payment Formula to Deal with Biased Selection.'' In *Advances In Health Economics and Health Services Research* 6, eds. R. M. Scheffler and L. F. Rossiter, 101–122. Greenwich, CT: JAI Press, 1985.

Luft, H. S. ''Competition and Regulation.'' *Medical Care* 23 (1985a): 383–400.

Luft, H. S. *Health Maintenance Organizations: Dimensions of Performance*. New York: John Wiley and Sons, Inc., 1981.

Luft, H. S. ''HMOs: Friends or Foes?'' *Business and Health* 3 (December 1985b): 5–10.

Luft, H. S. ''Health Maintenance Organizations and the Rationing of Medical Care.'' *Health and Society* 60 (1982): 268–306.

Luft, H. S. ''How Do Health Maintenance Organizations Achieve Their Savings?'' *The New England Journal of Medicine* 298 (1978): 1336–1343.

Luft, H. S. and S. C. Maerki. ''The Competitive Potential of Hospitals and Their Neighbors.'' *Contemporary Policy Issues* 3 (1985): 89–102.

Luft, H. S., and R. H. Miller. ''Patient Self-Selection in a Competitive Health Care System.'' *Health Affairs* 7 (1988): 97–119.

Luft, H. S., J. C. Robinson, D. W. Garnick, R. G. Hughes, S. J. McPhee, S. S. Hunt, and J. Showstack. ''Hospital Behavior in a Local Market Context.'' *Medical Care Review* 43 (1986): 217–251.

Luft, H. S., J. B. Trauner, and S. C. Maerki. ''Adverse Selection in a Large, Multi-Option Health Benefits Program: A Case Study of the California Public Employees' Retirement System.'' In *Advances in Health Economics and Health Services Research* 6, eds. R. M. Scheffler and L. F. Rossiter, 197–230. Greenwich, CT: JAI Press, 1985.

Luft, H. S., S. C. Maerki, and J. B. Trauner. ''The Competitive Effects of Health Maintenance Organizations: Another Look at the Evidence from Hawaii, Rochester and Minneapolis/St. Paul.'' *Journal of Health Politics, Policy and Law* 10 (1986): 625–658.

Luke, R. D., and M. A. Thomson. ''Utilization of Within Hospital Services: A Study of the Effects of Two Forms of Group Practice.'' *Medical Care* 17 (1980): 219–227.

Manning, W. G., A. Leibowitz, G. A. Goldberg, W. H. Rogers, and J. P. Newhouse. ''A Controlled Trial of the Effect of a Prepaid Group Practice on Use of Services.'' *The New England Journal of Medicine* 310 (1984): 1505–1510.

Manning, W. G., J. P. Newhouse, and J. W. Ware. ''The Status of Health in Demand Estimation; or, Beyond Excellent, Good, Fair, and Poor.'' In *Economic Aspects of Health*, ed. V. R. Fuchs, 143–184. Washington, DC: National Bureau of Economic Research, 1982.

Marcus, A. C., and J. F. Stone. ''Mode of Payment and Identification With a Regular Doctor.'' *Medical Care* 22 (1984): 647–657.

Marion Digest. *Managed Care Digest*. Kansas City, MO: Marion, 1990.

Marion. *Managed Care Digest: PPO Edition*. Kansas City, MO: Marion Laboratories, Inc., 1989.

McCall, N., E. D. Jay, and R. West. ''Access and Satisfaction in the Arizona Health Care Cost Containment System.'' *Health Care Financing Review* 11 (1989): 63–77.

McCall, N., and H. S. Wai. *An Analysis of the Use of Medicare Services by the Continuously Enrolled Aged.* Menlo Park, CA: SRI International, 1981.

McClure, W. "On Broadening the Definition of and Removing Barriers to a Competitive Health Care System." *Journal of Health Politics, Policy and Law* 3 (1978): 303–327.

McClure, W. "On the Research Status of Risk-Adjusted Capitation Rates." *Inquiry* 21 (1984): 205–213.

McCombs, J. S., J. D. Kasper and G. F. Riley. "Do HMOs Reduce Health Care Costs? A Multivariate Analysis of Two Medicare HMO Demonstration Projects." *Health Services Research* 25 (1990): 593–612.

McGuire, T. B. "Price and Membership in a Prepaid Group Medical Practice." *Medical Care* 19 (1981): 172–183.

McLaughlin, C. "HMO Growth and Hospital Expenses and Use: A Simultaneous-Equation Approach." *Health Services Research* 22 (1987): 183–205.

McLaughlin, C. "The Effect of HMOs on Overall Hospital Expenses: Is Anything Left After Correcting for Simultaneity and Selectivity?" *Health Services Research* 23 (1988): 421–441.

McLaughlin, C., J. C. Merrill, and A. J. Freed. "The Impact of HMO Growth on Hospital Costs and Utilization." In *Advances in Health Economics and Health Services Research*, 5, eds. R. M. Scheffler and L. F. Rossiter, 57–93. Greenwich, CT: JAI Press, 1984.

McMillan, A., J. Lubitz, and D. Russell. "Medicare Enrollment in Health Maintenance Organizations." *Health Care Financing Review* 8 (1987): 87–93.

Mechanic, D. "Consumer Choice Among Health Insurance Options." *Health Affairs* 8 (1990): 138–148.

Mechanic, D. "Cost Containment and the Quality of Medical Care: Rationing Strategies in an Era of Constrained Resources." *Health and Society* 63 (1985): 453–475.

Mechanic, D. "The Organization of Medical Practice and Practice Orientations Among Physicians in Prepaid and Non-Prepaid Primary Care Settings." *Medical Care* 13 (1975): 189–204.

Mechanic, D., N. Weiss, and P. D. Cleary. "The Growth of HMOs: Issues of Enrollment and Disenrollment." *Medical Care* 21 (1983): 338–347.

Meier, G. B., and J. Tillotson. *Physician Reimbursement and Hospital Use in HMOs.* Excelsior, MN: Interstudy, 1978.

Meier, G. B., and D. Aquilina. *Evaluating Health Maintenance Organizations: A Guide for Business, Labor and Coalitions.* Excelsior, MN.: InterStudy, 1982.

Mercer-Meidinger. *Evaluating Preferred Providers.* New York: William Mercer-Meidinger, 1985.

Merrill, J., and C. McLaughlin. "Competition Versus Regulation: Some Empirical Evidence." *Journal of Health Politics, Policy and Law* 10 (1986): 613–623.

Merrill, J., C. Jackson, and J. Reuter. "Factors that Affect the HMO Enrollment Decision: A Tale of Two Cities." *Inquiry* 22 (1985): 388–395.

Mirowsky, J., and C. E. Ross. "Patient Satisfaction and Visiting a Doctor: A Self-Regulating System." *Social Science and Medicine* 17 (1983): 1353–1361.

Mitchell, J. B. "Why Do Women Physicians Work Fewer Hours Than Men Physicians?" *Inquiry* 21 (1984): 361–368.

Moore, S. H., D. P. Martin, and W. C. Richardson. "Does the Primary-Care Gatekeeper

Control the Costs of Health Care?'' *The New England Journal of Medicine* 309: (1983): 1400–1404.

Morrisey, M. A., G. Gibson, and C. S. Ashley. ''Hospitals and Health Maintenance Organizations: An Analysis of the Minneapolis-St. Paul Experience.'' *Health Care Financing Review* 4 (1983): 59–69.

Mott, P. D. ''Hospital Utilization by Health Maintenance Organizations.'' *Medical Care* 24 (1986): 398–406.

Murray, J. P. ''A Comparison of Patient Satisfaction Among Prepaid and Fee-For-Service Patients.'' *Journal of Family Practice* 24 (1987): 203–207.

National Center for Health Statistics. ''Current Estimates from the National Health Interview Survey, United States, 1985.'' Hyattsville, MD: September 1986.

National Committee for Quality Assurance. *Overview and Status Report*. Washington, DC: National Committee, 1990.

Nelson, L., L. F. Rossiter, and K. Adamache. *Final Report on the Analysis of Aggregate Use and Cost Data From Medicare HMOs*. Contract No. 500–83–0047. Prepared for the Health Care Financing Administration. Washington, DC: Mathematica Policy Research, June, 1986.

Newcomer, R., C. Harrington, and A. Friedlob. ''Social Health Maintenance Organizations: Assessing Their Initial Experience.'' *Health Services Research* 25 (1990): 425–454.

Newhouse, J. P. ''Rate Adjusters for Medicare Under Capitation.'' *Health Care Financing Review* (Supplement, 1986): 45–55.

Newhouse, J. P., W. B. Schwartz, A. P. Williams, and C. Witsberger. ''Are Fee-For-Service Costs Increasing Faster Than HMO Costs?'' *Medical Care* 23 (1985): 962–966.

Oberg, C. N., C. L. Polich, and L. Kehn. *1987 Medicaid and HMO Data Book*. Excelsior, MN: InterStudy, 1987.

Oberg, C. N., and C. L. Polich. *Medicaid: Entering the Third Decade*. Excelsior, MN.: InterStudy, 1986.

Paley, W., and T. Bickman. *Report of Conference on Extending HMO Prepayment to Rural Areas*. Cloverack, NY: Caldwell B. Esselstyn Foundation, 1979.

Parker, M., C. L. Polich, L. R. Fischer, W. Pastor, H. Krulewitch, L. Pitt, P. Olson, and K. Korn. *The Provision of Home Care Services Through Health Maintenance Organizations*. Excelsior, MN.: InterStudy, 1988.

Peres, A. ''Is the HMO Act Good for Employers?'' *Business and Health* 5 (February 1988): 8–13.

Perspectives. ''Preferred Providers Proliferate.'' *Washington Report on Medicine and Health* (June 20, 1983): 3.

Polich, C. L., L. H. Iversen, and C. N. Oberg. ''HMOs as Providers of Health Services to the Elderly.'' *Clinical Report on Aging* 1 (1987a).

Polich, C. L., L. H. Iversen, and C. N. Oberg. *Risky Business: An Examination of TEFRA Risk HMOs and Their Risk Contracting Experience*. Excelsior, MN: InterStudy, 1987b.

''Poll Shows Mood to Spend on Health.'' *Medical Benefits* 7 (October 30, 1990): 2–3.

Porell, F. W., C. P. Tompkins, and W. M. Turner. ''Alternative Configurations for Medicare Payments to Health Maintenance Organizations.'' *Health Care Financing Review* 11 (1990): 17–30.

Powell, F. W., and W. M. Turner. "Biased Selection Under an Experimental Enrollment and Marketing Medicare HMO Broker." *Medical Care* 28 (1990): 604–615.

Price, J. R., J. W. Mays, and G. R. Trapnell. "Stability in the Federal Employees Health Benefits Program." *Journal of Health Economics* 2 (1983): 207–223.

Price, J. R., and J. W. Mays. "Selection and the Competitive Standing of Health Plans in a Multiple-Choice, Multiple-Insurer Market." *Advances in Health Economics and Health Services Research* 6, eds. R. M. Scheffler and L. F. Rossiter, 127–148. Greenwich, CT: JAI Press, 1985.

Ramsdell, J. W. "Physician Reimbursement for Services to HMO-Sponsored Patients: An Academic Model." *Medical Care* 23 (1985): 1315–1321.

Rayner, G. "HMOs in the USA and Britain: A New Prospect for Health Care." *Social Science and Medicine* 27 (1988): 305–320.

Rice, T., J. Gabel, and G. de Lissovoy. "PPOs: The Employer's Perspectives." *Journal of Health Politics, Policy and Law* 14 (1989): 367–382.

Rice, T., G. de Lissovoy, J. Gabel, and D. Ermann. "The State of PPOs: Results From a National Survey." *Health Affairs* 4 (1985): 25–39.

Rice, T. H. "The Impact of Changing Medicare Reimbursement Rates on Physician-Induced Demand." *Medical Care* 21 (1983): 803–815.

Riley, G., E. Rabey, and J. Kasper. "Biased Selection and Regression Toward the Mean in Three Medicare HMO Demonstrations: A Survival Analysis of Enrollees and Disenrollees." *Medical Care* 27 (1989): 337–351.

Robertson, W. O. "Costs of Diagnostic Tests: Estimates by Health Professionals." *Medical Care* 21 (1980): 556–559.

Rolph, E., P. Ginsburg, and S. Hosek. "Regulation of Preferred Provider Arrangements." *Health Affairs* 6 (1987): 46–60.

Roos, L. L. "Issues in Studying Ancillary Services." *Social Science and Medicine* 16 (1982): 1583–1590.

Rosenbach, M. L., B. S. Harrow, and S. Hurdle. "Physician Participation in Alternative Health Plans." *Health Care Financing Review* 9 (1988): 63–79.

Ross, M. H. "Rural Health Care—Is Prepayment a Solution?" *Public Health Reports* 90, No. 4 (July/August 1975): 293–302.

Rothert, M. L., D. R. Rovner, A. S. Elstein, G. B. Holzman, M. M. Holmes, and M. M. Ravitch. "Differences in Medical Referral Decisions for Obesity Among Family Practitioners, General Internists and Gynecologists." *Medical Care* 22 (1984): 42–55.

Rowland, D., and B. Lyons. "Mandatory HMO Care for Milwaukee's Poor." *Health Affairs* 6 (1987): 87–100.

Schaffer, W. A., F. D. Rollo, and C. A. Holt. "Falsification of Clinical Credentials by Physicians Applying for Ambulatory Staff Privileges." *New England Journal of Medicine* 318 (1988): 356–358.

Scheiber, G. J. "Health Expenditures in Major Industrialized Countries, 1960–87." *Health Care Financing Review* 11 (1990): 159–167.

Scitovsky, A., N. McCall, and L. Benham. "Factors Affecting the Choice Between Two Prepaid Plans." *Medical Care* 16 (1978): 660–681.

Shelton, N. "Competitive Contingencies in Selective Contracting for Hospital Services." *Medical Care Review* 46 (1989): 271–293.

Sloss, E. M., E. B. Kuler, R. H. Brook, B. H. Goldberg, and J. P. Newhouse. "Effect of a Health Maintenance Organization on Physiologic Health.'' *Annals of Internal Medicine* 106 (1987): 130.

Sox, H. C., I. Margulies, and C. H. Sox. ''Psychologically Mediated Effects of Diagnostic Tests.'' *Annals of Internal Medicine* 95 (1981): 680–685.

Spitz, B., and J. Abramson. ''Competition, Capitation, and Case Management: Barriers to Strategic Reform.'' *The Milbank Quarterly* 65 (1987): 348–370.

Stross, J. K., R. G. Hiss, C. M. Watts, W. K. Davis, and R. McDonald. ''Continuing Education in Pulmonary Disease for Primary-Care Physicians. *American Review of Respiratory Disorders* 127 (1983): 739–746.

''Survey Finds Elderly Highly Satisfied with Kaiser Portland's Medicare Plus Program.'' *Group Health News* 25 (1984): 11–12.

Sutton, H. ''Community Rating: An Historical Perspective.'' *Business and Health* 3 (July-August 1986): 41–44.

Tanzer, J., and J. Nudelman. ''Medicare and HMOs: A Marriage of Convenience?'' *Business and Health* 4 (August 1987): 34–36.

Tessler, R., and D. Mechanic. ''Factors Affecting the Choice Between Prepaid Group Practice and Alternative Insurance Programs.'' *Millbank Memorial Fund Quarterly* 54 (1975): 149–172.

Thomas, D. R., and K. M. Davis. ''Physician Awareness of Cost Under Prospective Reimbursement Systems.'' *Medical Care* 25 (1987): 181–184.

Thomas, J. W., R. Lichtenstein, L. Wyszewianski, and S. E. Berki. ''Increasing Medicare Enrollment in HMOs: The Need for Capitation Rates Adjusted for Health Status.'' *Inquiry* 20 (1983): 227–239.

Tierney, W. M., M. E. Miller, and C. J. McDonald. ''The Effect on Test Ordering of Informing Physicians of the Charges for Outpatient Diagnostic Tests.'' *The New England Journal of Medicine* 322 (1990): 1499–1504.

Topping, S. and M. D. Fottler. ''Improved Stakeholder Management: The Key to Revitalizing the HMO Movement.'' *Medical Care Review* 47 (1990): 365–393.

Traska, M. ''What Every Employer Needs to Know About HMOs.'' *Business and Health* 7 (June 1989): 18–29.

U.S. Congress. House Committee on Energy and Commerce. *Health Maintenance Organization Amendments of 1988: Report to Accompany H.R. 3235.*

U.S. Department of Health, Education, and Welfare: Office of Health Maintenance Organizations. *National Census of Prepaid Health Plans*. Washington, DC: 1980.

U.S. Department of Health, Education, and Welfare: Office of Health Maintenance Organizations. *National Census of Prepaid Health Plans*. Washington, DC: 1979.

U.S. Department of Health, Education, and Welfare: Office of Health Maintenance Organizations. *National Census of Prepaid Health Plans*. Washington, DC: 1978.

Van Hook, R. T. ''The Challenge of Rural Health.'' *Business and Health* 6 (December 1988): 4–6.

Varner, T., and J. Christy. ''Consumer Information Needs in a Competitive Healthcare Environment.'' *Health Care Financing Review* (Supplement 1986): 99–104.

Viau, S. *PPOs: The State of the Art*. Washington, DC: Health Publishing Ventures, 1983.

Wagner, E. H. and T. Bledsoe. ''The Rand Health Insurance Experiment and HMOs.'' *Medical Care* 28 (1990): 191–200.

Wallack, S. S., C. P. Tompkins, and L. Gruenberg. ''A Plan for Rewarding Efficient HMOs.'' *Health Affairs* 7 (1988): 80–96.

Ware, J. E., et al. ''Effects of Differences in Quality of Care on Patient Satisfaction Solution.'' *Proceedings, Seventeenth Annual Conference on Research in Medical Education*. Washington, DC: 1978.

Ware, J. E., R. H. Brook, and W. H. Rogers. ''Comparison of Health Outcomes at Health Maintenance Organizations With Those of Fee-For-Service Care.'' *The Lancet* (1986): 1017–1022.

Ware, J. E., R. H. Brook, and W. H. Rogers. *Medicaid Satisfaction Surveys, 1977–1980: A Report of the Prepaid Health Research, Evaluation, and Development Project*. Sacramento, CA: California State Department of Health Services, 1981.

Welch, W. P. ''Medicare Capitation Payments to HMOs In Light of Regression Toward the Mean in Health Care Costs.'' In *Advances in Health Economics and Health Services Research* 6, eds. R. M. Scheffler and L. F. Rossiter, 75–96. Greenwich, CT: JAI Press, 1985.

Welch, W. P. ''The New Structure of Individual Practice Associations.'' *Journal of Health Politics, Policy and Law* 12 (1987): 723–739.

Welch, W. P., R. G. Frank, and P. Diehr. ''Health Care Costs in Health Maintenance Organizations: Correcting for Self-Selection.'' In *Advances in Health Economics and Health Services Research* 5, eds. R. M. Scheffler and L. F. Rossiter, 95–128. Greenwich, CT: JAI Press, 1984.

Welch, W. P., A. L. Hillman, and M. V. Pauly. ''Toward New Typologies for HMOs.'' *The Milbank Quarterly* 68 (1990): 221–243.

Welch, W. P., and M. E. Miller. ''Mandatory Enrollment in Medicaid: The Issue of Freedom of Choice.'' *The Milbank Quarterly* 66 (1988): 618–639.

Wennberg, J. E., and A. Gittelsohn. ''Variations in Medical Care Among Small Areas.'' *Scientific American* 246 (1982): 120–134.

Wilensky, G. R., and L. F. Rossiter. ''Patient Self-Selection in HMOs.'' *Health Affairs* 5 (1986): 66–80.

Wolinsky, F., and W. Marder. ''Spending Time With Patients: The Impact of Organizational Structure on Medical Practice.'' *Medical Care* 20 (1982): 1051.

Wollstadt, L. J., S. Shapiro, and T. W. Bice. ''Disenrollment from a Prepaid Group Practice: An Actuarial and Demographic Description.'' *Inquiry* 15 (1978): 142–150.

Wouters, A., and J. Hester. ''Patient Choice of Providers in a Preferred Provider Organization.'' *Medical Care* 26 (1988): 240–255.

Wrightson, C. W. *HMO Rate Setting and Financial Strategy*. Ann Arbor, MI: Health Administration Press, 1990.

Wyszewianski, L., J.R.C. Wheller, and A. Donabedian. Market-Oriented Cost-Containment and Quality of Care.'' *Milbank Memorial Fund Quarterly* 60 (1982): 518–550.

Yelin, E. H., M. A. Shearn, and W. V. Epstein. ''Health Outcomes for a Chronic Disease in Prepaid Group Practice and Fee-For-Service Settings.'' *Medical Care* 24 (1986): 236–247.

Yett, D. E., W. Der, R. L. Ernst, and J. W. Hay. ''Physician Pricing and Health Insurance Reimbursement.'' *Health Care Financing Review* 5 (1983): 69–80.

# Index

## About the Author

**PERRY MOORE** is Dean of the College of Liberal Arts of Wright State University. His previous work on health care cost containment was published by the International Personnel Management Association.